"In this book, Julia Aziz masterfully distills out the wisdom of her own childbearing experiences and offers readers a treasure trove of deep and simple gems of inspiration for navigating the journey into and through motherhood. This is not *a way of doing* it, rather *a way of being present* to one's self and the fleeting moments of family life. With reminders to slow down, experiment, let go and trust yourself... this book is essential reading for anyone who is a mother, has been mothered or is about to embark on the journey of motherhood."

– Carrie Contey, PhD, internationally recognized parenting coach and founder of Evolve

"I know some midwives who've said for years they wanted to write about the parallels between life and labor. I think when they see this book they will slap their thighs and say, somebody did it!"

- Pam England, author of *Birthing From Within*

"From her own unique and varied childbearing experiences, Julia Aziz learned much beyond what labor and birth can be like; she guides us through her musings on the lessons gained from her labors—about life as a woman, life partner, mother, and human being. This engaging book, told in her personable style and warm voice, relates how she was transformed, and her pithy wisdom helps us see how we also may be transformed by life's unpredictable adventures."

– Penny Simkin, author of *The Birth Partner: A Complete Guide to Childbirth for Dads, Doulas, and All Other Labor Companions*, co-founder of DONA International (formerly Doulas of North America)

"Here's a book that lets us parents know we aren't alone with our worries, doubts, fears—and we don't have to be ashamed or overwhelmed by them, either."
> – Lenore Skenazy, author of *Free-Range Kids*

"In *Lessons of Labor*, Julia Aziz offers a vulnerable perspective of personal growth, wisdom of the body, and a lesson in surrender."
> – Latham Thomas, author of *Mama Glow: A Hip Guide to Your Fabulous Abundant Pregnancy*

"This excellent book will help new mothers process their birth experiences and gain valuable insights about their transformation into motherhood."
> – Diana West, IBCLC, co-author of the 8th edition of La Leche League International's *The Womanly Art of Breastfeeding*

"*Lessons of Labor* holds so many pearls of wisdom that can only be gained by trusting the process of childbirth and parenting. Julia's story reflects the universal nature of mothering from the small details to the big picture. I will be recommending this book to all my clients, regardless of how many times they've given birth. It was a joy to read."
> – Sarita Bennett, DO, CPM, osteopathic family practice physician, midwife, vice president of the Midwives Alliance of North America

"In *Lessons of Labor*, Julia Aziz offers readers the hope that through parenting we can really come to know and trust our own selves. The stories and lessons shared take the reader through explorations of parenting, partnering and self–the flaws, the feelings and the idea that the journey of parenting can be our best teacher. Throughout the book, Aziz offers comfort to a tired mama soul and inspiration toward becoming the most connected and joyful self we can possibly be at any given moment, all the while knowing that new moments and new lessons just keep on coming!"

> – Bernadette Noll, author of *Slow Family Living*

"Aziz's words echoed my own lessons as a young mother. *Lessons of Labor* feels like a present to my own daughter because this is what I want her to understand about labor, motherhood, and the gifts it can bring. An inspirational read for mothers, birth professionals, and those that care for them!"

> – Amy Gilliland, PhD, DONA International Birth Doula Trainer

"Take the time to savor this book; it will remind you to appreciate and to trust the ever-changing and individual needs of each member of your family as well as yourself."

> – Phyllis Klaus, MFT, LMSW, psychotherapist, co-author of *Your Amazing Newborn, Mothering the Mother,* and *Bonding: Building the Foundations of Secure Attachment and Independence,* co-founder of DONA International

"In her book, Aziz brings you beautifully through the journey of pregnancy and into the life thereafter."

> – Shawn Tassone, MD, PhD, author of *Spiritual Pregnancy: Develop, Nurture & Embrace the Journey to Motherhood*

"Julia Aziz is a wonderful storyteller. The stories she shares of the transformative experiences of pregnancy, birth, and of mothering are both intimately personal and touchingly universal. They connect us as women, as parents, and as human beings."

– Barbara Wilson-Clay, BS, IBCLC, FILCA, author of *The Breastfeeding Atlas*

Lessons of Labor

One Woman's Self-Discovery
Through Birth & Motherhood

Julia S. Aziz

Health & Fitness: Pregnancy and Childbirth
Family & Relationship: Parenting - Motherhood
Self-Help: Personal Growth - General

Copyright 2015 by MSI Press

For information, contact
MSI Press
1760-F Airline Highway, #203
Hollister, CA 95023

Library of Congress Control Number 2014942193

ISBN: 978-1-933455-92-1

Contents

For Patrick, Kaleb, Jeremiah, Marisa, and Obie

I never had to learn to love you. That part comes easy.

Introduction

Before giving birth for the first time, I was warned that labor would be the most painful physical experience I would ever endure, but no one ever told me I would be entering into battle with my mind. No one explained that the pain of labor was just as much about facing my inner demons and giving up the pretense of control as it was about physical discomfort. I also didn't know that I would keep learning from the experience for the rest of my life.

This book is not a manual for having a "successful" natural birth or for becoming the ultimate Zen mother. Though you may have been searching for such a guide, I do not think you need one. I offer you the stories of my birth and early motherhood experiences to share the learning I received through this incredible rite of passage. Instead of teaching you how to labor or how to live your life, my reflections are meant to ignite your curiosity about your own labor as an opportunity for self-discovery. More than anything, I hope this book inspires you to trust deeply that your life experience is your greatest teacher.

A Little about Me

I have been lucky, very much so. I did not encounter any truly unmanageable complications during my pregnancies or births. I had a supportive husband and adequate health care. The struggles I encountered derived mostly from a low-level anxiety I have lived with my whole life. It's a default mode of functioning when I'm under duress or facing something new. I used to try to hide my worry and tension, but now I see that I can be of more service to both myself and others if I bring these old patterns into the light. From counseling countless mothers and sharing stories with friends, I have realized that I am not alone. Most of us get a little crazy sometimes; we just get crazy about different things. This book is for women who hunger for some perspective and encouragement that won't fuel their fears or increase their self-imposed pressure.

I have three children, the first born in the hospital and the second two at home. Before any of them were to enter my life, I became pregnant for the first time but lost that very small baby in an early miscarriage. That first birth and loss is part of my story, too, and it offers its own wisdom. For this reason, I share it with you in these pages as well.

Why We Can Learn Something from Giving Birth

All our life experiences, if viewed through the lens of open curiosity, can be used for personal growth. In the regular, everyday world, we perceive change slowly. Days or months can pass with nothing seemingly new, but with more intense situations, everything we normally experience in our interior world arrives in a rush. My whole life story—every theme and every emotion—has seemingly been played out in fast and hard encounters like a ten-day meditation retreat, a five-week road trip, or twelve hours of labor. What I have seen and learned there is accessible, raw, and meaningful. The memories are touchstones to return to again and again.

Birth and death are, by their nature, the most intense experiences we will have in our lifetime. Most of us cannot remember our own births, and we can't tell the story of our deaths. So, giving birth to another human being, in my opinion, is about as fundamental a transformation as we can hope to experience consciously. Not only do we become Mother through this difficult passage, but we also experience the loss of the greatest intimacy possible—that of one person living *inside* another. It is as mundane as it gets but also uniquely amazing and profound.

Women anticipate labor with every emotion there is, from eagerness and joy to anxiety and dread, often with good doses of impatience or ambivalence as well. Many women yearn to have the perfect birth and write birth plans in an attempt to safeguard their way. I, too, wrote a birth plan the first time around. I hoped it would protect me from everything I feared and from the unknown in general. The plan would demonstrate how informed I was and would help me stay in control. Only during that first labor did I realize how having a baby is nothing if not an experience of complete loss of control. This is not something modern women enjoy all that much. So much of our pre-baby lives are spent making choices and decisions, deciding what we want and figuring out how to get it. Having a child is nothing like that!

For many of us, once we've given birth, the urge to share our stories is strong, but in the surge of activity involved in taking care of a newborn baby, these stories soon fade into the distance. They are remembered with less and less detail and eventually less emotional charge. Soon, they become quick summaries, judged "good" if they matched our desires and "bad" if they didn't.

There may be something more to our stories than just whether we had a good or bad birth experience, though. We might consider questions beyond whether or not everything went the way we wanted. Instead, we might ask what these birth stories tell us about ourselves. What meaning can we find in the particular way we came face to face with pain, with the unknown, and with the delivery of new life into this world? How might we use this experience in the future? Can it teach us something about how we mother our children or about who we are becoming in this next phase of our lives?

The Book

Lessons of Labor is divided into four parts (Babies 1, 2, 3, and Miscarriage), each consisting of multiple short chapters. The chapters begin with excerpts from my birth stories, all of which were recorded within hours of the actual experiences. After each excerpt, a simple but relevant insight is offered. These "lessons of labor" are followed by essays that reflect on how the challenges of birthing are analogous to the personal growth opportunities of early motherhood. While the birth story excerpts follow the sequential experience of labor, the discussions after each lesson were written at different times, and they span the past decade of my life.

To be clear, it's not as if I gave birth, learned some life lessons, and then lived happily or wisely ever after.

Sometimes, I was inspired while breathing deeply through a contraction; other times, I discovered something new when I looked back in retrospect. In the big picture, I have been learning these lessons since my own birth, and I relearn them every time I fall off course. Like a hidden curriculum for my life, they lie beneath the surface of both my mundane and extraordinary moments.

For You, the Reader

The lessons in this book are not prescriptions for living. They are reminders, little lamps on in the house next door that let you know you are not alone. I hope to remind you of what you already know but maybe have forgotten for a time. I hope to inspire you to look at your own life, no matter what it encompasses, as an opportunity to learn and to love, to heal and to grow. Becoming a mother is part of the journey of discovery, one of adventure, pain, love, and surprises.

Above all, I hope you become your own best advisor in the birthing process, in parenting, and in living. May this book remind you to dive deeper into life, to reflect and learn as you go, and to make the most out of whatever is born to you.

Julia S. Aziz

BABY 1

Birthing for the First Time: The Lesson of "I Can Survive"

Julia S. Aziz

Labor Begins When Other Labors Cease

The day of my first son's birth was one of those early spring days that make me happy to live in Austin, Texas. The sun was shining, the flowers were in bloom, and I was feeling some mild but noticeable cramps. I felt eager, open, and fully welcoming of my baby as I walked through the neighborhood, telling my belly, "What a beautiful day to be born!" As with most new experiences, I started off with high hopes and great determination. After a few hours, I began my preparations: making sure my bags were packed, adding essential items like a toothbrush and contact lens solution, preparing a light meal that would be easy to digest, and otherwise doing a lot of stuff that would later prove mostly unnecessary.

After a while, I began to feel agitated. I wanted to get everything done, but my detail-oriented mind was slowly being overtaken by my body's strong messages. I was losing concentration, unable to focus on the thoughts in my head. I would reach for more CDs to put in my hospital bag and then start looking in the closet, wondering if I should bring a bathrobe. Then, a contraction would hit, and I would walk around in circles, concerned that I wasn't going to be able to finish either task because it just hurt too much. I wanted to complete what I had begun, but my body had other plans.

There is freedom in saying, "I've done enough," even when the job is somewhat flawed or unfinished.

Growing up through school and into adulthood, I was taught to finish what I started. It felt good to work hard and then relax when the work was done. Then, motherhood set in, and as a mother, knowing how to finish hasn't been nearly as important as knowing when to quit.

At the end of each day, until our lives are over, some tasks will be left undone. Since true completion is often unattainable, I must learn to discern when I have dedicated enough effort to a project—to say, "Good enough!" and move on. Sometimes another need is more pressing, or sometimes I just want a break. Whatever the reason, I am learning that being done can be more about my state of mind and less about the state my work is in.

The lesson of letting go of a task before it meets an ideal standard has been hard won for me. I used to be someone who could dive into a project, focus intently, and work until the end appeared. Take packing up a household for a move, for instance. In my life before parenthood, I would spend a day packing boxes and driving a truck back and forth across town, and then I would feel tired and complete when it was all over. But moving with small children? It wasn't like that at all. I had to get tasks done in small increments of time, and the process was often sloppy. If the baby took an unexpected nap, I would grab some boxes and pack up the dishes until he woke up. If the kids were playing outside, I would call the utility company and wait on hold while making lunch. In the end, some things never made it into boxes but instead ended up in multiple piles in the car. It took about thirty trips across town and weeks of haphazard living, but we still arrived where we needed to be (and then took our time—a year?—to unpack once we got there).

While I often miss the satisfaction of completion, now I get to experience the freedom of letting go. Transitioning back to regular work with three small children has given me plenty of opportunities for this experience. I can be in the middle of something pressing, something that would feel completed if I just stayed an extra half hour to finish up, but my babysitter has to leave, or maybe I need to nurse the baby. Whatever it is, I have to let go of the incomplete project, lock the office, and go home. The more I leave work unfinished, the more I experience a certain freedom that comes with giving up. I feel free not because I am done but because I am not done! I can *choose* to leave, instead of being held prisoner by my desire for the perfect finale.

Julia S. Aziz

The Priority of the Present

Finally, I recognized that my will could no longer compete with my body. I put the half-cooked meal in the freezer and the mostly packed bags by the door. I needed to direct my full attention to labor. I moved slowly around the house, resting over the arms of couches and chairs, breathing deeply, and moaning quietly. Without the pressure of tasks to accomplish, I was able to notice that my contractions had progressed from the menstrual-like cramping sensation of before. They were now much stronger and more substantial. Something was really happening here.

When necessity pulls me into the present, I know exactly what matters.

One of the blessings of labor for me was the inability to attend to everyday minutiae. The sensations of my body became so powerful that my usual multi-tasking mindset started to fade into the distance. Though the mental chatter continued, it wasn't in command anymore. I was able to access a deeper focus, the same mental focus that arises when a crisis occurs. All the usual concerns are available, like background music, but the foreground is highly charged and almost all-encompassing.

When I was about eight months into my second pregnancy, I took my two-year-old son to an outdoor festival. It was a fun and stimulating late-spring celebration with lots of live music to dance to and crafts booths to browse. I was enjoying being with friends but was also somewhat distracted by hunger, fatigue, and the usual third-trimester aches and pains. When a group of us stopped to chat around a fountain, I asked a friend to watch my toddler while I made yet another visit to the restroom. When I returned a few minutes later, my friend and I stared at each other in shock, both asking where my son had gone. She anxiously told me that she thought he was with me, since after I had walked away he had followed me to the bathroom. I spun around in an instant and headed first for the outside gate to the road, yelling his name. Despite my heavy, aching belly, I ran through the festival, asking everyone if they had seen a toddler boy alone. Within a few minutes, I spotted him. My son had been found by a kind AmeriCorps volunteer, and together they had been searching for me. We ran into each other's arms, my son crying out his own name, as if to say, "How could you have forgotten me?" We hugged and cried and hugged some more, both of us finding great relief in this moment of reunion.

Those few minutes were so terrifying that all I could focus on was finding my son. I had been single-minded in purpose, and it was hours before the intensity of my concentration relaxed. It wasn't until later that afternoon that I even noticed the strong (though not dangerous) Braxton-Hicks contractions that had come on after all the running and adrenaline. My gratitude for having my son back far outweighed any physical discomfort I had to endure.

Even better than waiting for a crisis or a baby to be born is when I can consciously choose to give my whole self to what really matters in the present moment. This morning, for instance, I found myself racing from one thing to the next like the proverbial headless chicken: speeding to the bank and the store, nursing the baby every twenty minutes in an attempt to induce sleep, rotating three loads of laundry necessitated by various toileting accidents and diaper explosions, installing a car seat, and making arrangements for a job interview. Then, my son asked me to put on a puppet show.

"Please, just for a minute. Please, Mommy."

I didn't want to. I wanted to just keep going and going. Today, though, I looked at my son and saw myself through his eyes. I saw that he could see my frenzy and just wanted my presence. I realized in that moment that I wanted to be the kind of mom who could put aside the chores to play with her child. So, I did it. I put on a very silly improvisational puppet show, listened to my child's laughter, and took a few moments to enjoy being together.

Then, I went back to my list of three million things. Of course! Yet, if one blessing of labor (or a crisis) is knowing the clear priority in the present moment, maybe I can practice receiving that blessing in ordinary time, if only for a minute.

Julia S. Aziz

Asking for Help

The next step was to call the midwife who would be acting as my doula. Though I knew and trusted Meredith fully, the act of calling her was preceded by much ambivalent deliberation. Was it too early to call? Would I be wasting her time if I asked her to come now? I didn't want to bother her or interfere in her day if it wasn't necessary, but my labor was becoming more demanding. I wanted someone who had seen it before to guide me. So, I gave over to my need and called her. Happily, she offered to come over to my house and see how I was doing.

I can ask for what I need.
I can receive what is given.

Why is it so hard to ask for help? I encountered the same tendency to doubt the legitimacy of my needs in all three of my labors, to such a degree with the third that I almost ended up delivering my own baby! In our culture, a strong woman is often defined as one who can take care of herself. There is a certain pride to be found in this sort of independence, but pregnancy and motherhood have been knocking down this idol for me. Not since my own childhood have I felt so dependent. I have had to depend on my healthcare providers, depend deeply on my husband (so long, traditional feminist ideals!), and depend on the wisdom and generosity of my friends and family.

I will always remember arriving home from the hospital a few days after giving birth for the first time. I had been amped up since my baby was born and had not slept at all. My feeling of manic exhaustion escalated when it came time to feed the baby. I had been struggling with breastfeeding since the beginning but had persevered under the guidance of seasoned nurses at the hospital. They had propped my arms up on at least five different pillows and patiently held my baby's head so that he could properly latch. Suddenly, I was home and had no idea how to nurse on my own. In some primal way, I felt like my baby would starve to death if I didn't immediately give him the milk he cried for. When my multiple attempts to latch the baby were unsuccessful, I called a friend who lived nearby to ask if she could come over and help. She came right away, without hesitation. She helped me create a comfortable space to nurse in the house and taught me how to feed the baby while lying down in bed. Taking a deep breath of relief, I told her how grateful I was for her calm presence and sensible advice. It all seemed so urgent and essential to me, and yet, as she reminded me, it was really just a small favor to ask of her.

As I work on letting go of the pressure to be self-sufficient, I see that accepting help allows others true entrance into my life, creating the stronger community that I always longed to have. After that first birth, a group of dear friends took turns bringing dinner to our house. I didn't realize in advance what a great gift this would be. With less time needed for food preparation, my husband and I were given more time to learn how to take care of our newborn and to adjust to being parents. Each meal, so lovingly prepared, reminded us that we were supported and cared for. It felt like our little family was truly part of a greater whole.

When I gave birth to my second and third babies, friends asked me for a list of names so they could invite people to bring meals again. Both times, I gave the names not just of other friends but of some acquaintances and colleagues too—anyone who had mentioned that they wanted to help out in some way. I decided that inviting people to bring food was not the same as obligating them to do so. I reminded myself that if someone wanted to give, I didn't need to politely decline; it was okay to graciously receive. Both times, we received two months of daily home-cooked meals as a result of that extended network of generosity. The pride of independence was replaced with deep and lasting gratitude. In turn, now that I know how meaningful this gift can be, I rarely miss an opportunity to bring a new family a meal.

Julia S. Aziz

Trying Something New

Once the doula arrived, I was able to commit my whole self to the adventure of having a baby. I found a rhythm that involved pacing slowly around the flowering tree in the backyard, leaning on my husband for support, and resting between contractions. My body responded with the building momentum of active labor.

As the intensity grew, I began to struggle. I became restless, uncomfortable, and unable to find a good position during the contractions. The tree-circling was no longer working. Seeing my discomfort, the doula suggested I move into the shower. The water pounding on my back made an unmistakable difference. I was able to lean my weight onto my husband's arms and let the water beat down on me, a wonderful new sensation. All it took was that small change, and I was able to enter the zone again.

If it's not working, it may be time to try something new.

Parents and children may go through some trial and error before finding comfortable routines, but eventually we settle into a groove, finding our individual places in the family pattern. Once I get the hang of my part, a new challenge arises: I become attached to my way of doing things and sometimes forget that other possibilities exist. As needs and circumstances change, old habits may no longer serve me or my loved ones as well as they used to. It may take time to realize that what I am doing is no longer helpful, but once I see clearly, the best course of action is to try something new.

As I write this now, I am sitting in a hotel room in San Antonio, quietly editing while my daughter naps nearby in her port-a-crib. This morning, as we got ready to leave our house for the weekend, I found myself compelled to enter my autopilot mode for trip preparation. In this mode, I work quickly and efficiently, packing up the kids' and my belongings, putting together food for travel, and making sure the house is closed up. It used to take me many hours to prepare for a weekend getaway with the children, but over time, I developed a system that could get us out the door soon after breakfast. While this system was still effective in getting things done, it was starting to have some unfortunate side effects. Sometimes, I have been so absorbed in my desire for efficiency that I have started pressuring everyone around me. While I am urging the children out the door, my husband is often still packing his bag, and then discord ensues.

This morning as I began packing, I paused and considered how my impatience had been affecting the other people in my family. I decided I didn't want to create the tense energy of rushing, and maybe it would be better if I didn't play my old role today. Instead of speeding up, I could try slowing down. So I purposefully let go of my concern about what time we left the house. I finished all the preparations that needed to be done, and then I went outside to read a book. When the kids asked repeatedly to leave, I just told them they could play some more while daddy finished what he was doing. Guess what? We are here now, maybe a little later than I thought we would be, but with peace instead of conflict to start our vacation. The only change I had to make was to relax into my morning instead of pushing a process that wasn't finished yet.

There is usually more than one way to approach a situation. I just have to be willing to take notice and experiment. I don't need to force change on anyone else. Even when just one of us tries something new, the whole family pattern can come back into balance.

Julia S. Aziz

Facing Fear

Once I was ready to get out of the shower, the doula rec-ommended that we leave for the hospital. She checked my cer-vix, reassuring me that I was far enough along in the process to warrant a move to the final birthing destination. Before gathering all my belongings, I had a crisis of faith. How would I ever manage the pain of labor while sitting in the car for 30 minutes? At home, I could walk outside and bend over with every contraction, impossible activities for the front seat of a car. I even started to debate just staying home (my doula was a homebirth midwife, after all). Then, reason, or rather my husband's calm rationality, took over, and we decided to go with the plan already in place. Internally, I said to myself, "I can do this because I have to and because no one else can do it for me."

Sometimes, the only way past the hard stuff is through it.

When I am in a situation where there is no out, for a few moments I may feel trapped. If I break free of that fear, then I see that there is one thing I can do, and that is to face up to what's in front of me. There is a freedom in having only one viable course of action. I don't need to brainstorm, and I don't need to negotiate. There is nothing to fight and no-where to flee. There is just this: the clarity of knowing what

I have to do and a newfound strength to do it. This improbable freedom comes with surrendering to my place in the universe right here, right now. Knowing and accepting that I cannot escape my circumstances means I don't need to worry about anything. I can just follow the path in front of me even if it does look treacherous.

I will never forget the time when my twelve-week-old infant needed urgent medical care for an accidental injury that occurred in the middle of the night. When my husband lifted the baby up to check his diaper in the darkened nursery, the baby had lunged forward mid-air, and the racing ceiling fan had struck him somewhere in the vicinity of his head. The baby was crying loudly without pause, and we couldn't tell exactly where or how badly he was hurt. The pediatrician on-call told us to go to the emergency room immediately. I had a moment of panic ("I'm not strong enough to handle this!") before this same message came to me: I can do this because I have to. My husband and I rushed our baby to the closest hospital. He parked the car while I ran down the hallways with my infant son, whispering, "You're okay, you're okay, I love you."

We waited through a tense four hours in the ER waiting room. I held our baby in my arms, realizing just how thoroughly devoted I was to this fragile new life. I knew, deep in my bones, that if anything were to happen to him, my heart would never truly recover. I had no choice but to live through the fear, though. There was no avoiding the frantic rushing, the dread, or the waiting. Finally, my son was examined and, thankfully, found to have no lasting repercussions from the accident, just a bruise on his cheek.

We often think of babies as being vulnerable—to illness, to injury, to poor child-rearing—but new mothers are vulnerable, too. My heart has never been the same since I became a mother. Each child has taken a part of me into the world with him or her, a part that is as essential to my well-being as the rest of me, but what can I do? Hold my children so close that I suffocate them? Or instead, should I not let myself love them so much? It's not even possible with a love that immense. So, my heart stays open, and I go through both the easy and the hard parts that come with having children. Being a parent is a wild ride, and it takes great courage and a spirit of adventure. In the most challenging times, it helps to remember that there is only one course: living through what happens.

Julia S. Aziz

Change Happens

I got in the car and coped with those contractions much better than I imagined I would. They didn't feel as difficult to bear as they had felt at home even though I was forced to sit in a very uncomfortable position (that of a normal person in a passenger seat). Once I arrived at the hospital, though, BOOM! Wrenching pain surged with a vengeance. I had to stop and squat in the parking lot, the elevator, and the hallway as I made my way up to the labor and delivery room, where I would remain until my baby was born.

As the contractions grew stronger, I became flustered. I wanted to figure out what was going on in my body so I could somehow manage my labor, but just when I would find a rhythm with my breath or my movement, the contractions would get harder, or longer, or something would change. What was working before wouldn't work anymore. I was trying to mentally get ahead of the contractions when clearly my body was ahead of my mind. What I really needed was to observe more closely and perceive the changes as they occurred.

If there is one thing I can count on, it's change.

I remember the truth of the inevitability of change every time one of my children makes a developmental leap. Whether it's learning to roll over, taking first steps, or reading the words on a street sign, I am frequently taken off guard when

I see my child growing up. A part of me just wants to hold on to my babies, and that attachment to the past makes it hard for me to believe we have already moved into the future.

When my first child was only a year and a half old, he climbed out of his crib. My husband and I were talking in the living room when we heard a big thump. Next thing we knew, our son was toddling down the hallway. Convinced we could teach him to stay in his crib, we tried putting him in again. Thump! Again, he was out. This was a child who loved to move and cherished his freedom. So, with some apprehension, we took apart the crib, converting it into a toddler bed with a safety rail.

About two weeks later, this active boy fell off a short stool in a shoe store and broke his leg. Because of his heavy cast, he rolled off his new toddler bed that night and crashed onto the floor. (Did I mention that he had been surreptitiously taking off the toddler rail himself every night before sleep? He is not a big fan of restraints.) Concerned about him falling off his bed every night with an already broken limb, we decided to put his crib back together. Surely, this containment would keep him safe and allow him to sleep better. So, the next night, he was back in his crib. After saying goodnight, my husband and I went into the living room. Thump! Our son had managed to scale the side of his crib with a broken leg in a cast, and he had fallen down to the floor again. This only had to happen once, as we were finally convinced. The boy was done with his crib. Realizing that his will and strength had grown and that this new phase was real and irreversible, we arranged a futon mattress on the floor for him to sleep on. That way, our son could have his freedom without the potential for heavy-weighted falls in the night.

The most predictable part of parenthood is knowing that nothing will stay the same as it is right now. "Hold on!" I sometimes want to say. "Let me get a handle on this part first!" But, no, the world keeps spinning, and my children keep growing. I might as well, too.

Julia S. Aziz

Alone, in Good Company

My husband existed in the periphery of my focus. I knew that he was right there with me, rubbing my back, breathing with me, and sometimes supporting my entire weight as I squatted and squeezed his arms. I knew that he was in sync, unafraid, and altogether attentive. I also knew there was only so much he could do to help me. He could not take away my pain.

My doula, too, was incredible. She was perceptive, patient, and highly skilled. She consistently encouraged me but also stood back enough to let my husband and me share this intimate experience. Of course, she, also, could not have my baby for me.

As I labored in the hospital, I could hear conversations in the background. A nurse came in and made small talk about dinner. I found the topic bizarre. Who could think of such things at a time like this, when my body was being ripped apart from the inside out? But it was my body, not hers, and she was doing her best to be kind and unobtrusive. I had amazing support all around me, and, at the same time, my experience was a solitary one.

I am in this alone, and we are in this together.

I believed I would be able to labor and give birth without painkillers as long as no unforeseen complications occurred.

I had this confidence because so many women had gone through this pain before me. Even though they were not in the room with me, I took courage from knowing that if they could do it, so could I. It wasn't a contest to see how much pain I could take or how lucky I could be to avoid something terrible happening. It was just an inner longing to feel the entire physical experience of giving birth, the way my fore-mothers did throughout human history. I knew I couldn't control the process or outcome of my birth experience because there was always a chance I would need medical intervention for health or safety reasons. I could, however, choose how to approach the challenge of giving birth. I chose to be alone in the pain of labor, just like generations of women before me had been.

In some ways, I am always on my own. No one can live my life for me. In other ways, however, even as I am aware of my separateness, I know also that we are all alone together. When I am feeling isolated in my experience, it is valuable for me to remember that there are other people out there feeling the same way.

Recently, I told my neighbor, a new mother of a two-week-old baby, that seeing her light on at 2:30 a.m. made me smile. I had gone to the bathroom, having just nursed my daughter, and saw the reflection of her light through my window. Though I was tired and weary, I felt a little leap in my heart. Someone else was up in the middle of the night, nursing a baby! It was nice to think that we were in this together even while we were each alone in our own houses. Of all the countless, long nights I spent nursing my babies, alone in the midnight and early morning darkness, this was one of my favorites.

Resistance

Somehow, even though I was breathing through the contractions, staying upright and mobile, varying my position, receiving massages and emotional support, listening to calming music, and experiencing a healthy, safe, naturally progressing labor, I wasn't happy at all. I was furious. I could not get on top of the experience. I felt like I was at war with the contractions, and they were winning. They came at me like the pounding surf, over and over again, each one stronger and each one pulling my fighting attitude down with it. When I wasn't struggling to subdue my body, I was fiercely wishing to escape it.

This is the only moment I have. Resisting my experiences, even the really hard ones, won't make them go away. It will just make them harder.

I once heard a Buddhist teaching about learning to ride a horse as a metaphor for resistance. When I refuse to embrace a difficult challenge, they say it is like trying to ride a horse on top of another horse, instead of just learning to ride the first horse alone. How silly is that? Since the obstacle I am facing is demanding enough as is, adding on resistance (I don't want this!) provides no benefit.

Like most wisdom, this is something I can easily recognize when I pay attention to what I am doing. Noticing how

I make things harder for myself, I can consciously let go of some of my resistance. The hour before bedtime is a good example. When the three children are all safely tucked away at night, I can relax, finally free from all obligations. The hour just before, though, is full of responsibilities: cleaning, bathing, teeth brushing, helping with pajamas, reading stories, tucking in, helping with the bathroom, tucking in again, bringing water, tucking in again, and so on. Sometimes, bedtime feels like the finish line of a long race, and that last leg is the hardest.

The children are often still running gleeful circles around the house when the clock says they should be getting ready for bed. While I feel tired and want to slow down, they seem to be catching a second wind. I often want to erase this part of the day, this time when my energy is already low and the children still need so much assistance. My muscles clench in frustration as I try to herd the children toward their chores, and I start internally counting down the minutes until silence reigns. My resistant attitude just intensifies the bedtime battles, though. I start taking the last-minute requests and refusals to sleep personally, as if the children are purposefully trying to steal my downtime. What began as just a physically effortful hour becomes also an emotional struggle. I find myself straining to maintain a patient tone of voice while inwardly raging at the injustice of it all.

When I consciously release the resistance to my nighttime duties, I can choose to take a different approach. I can just stay with the moment, doing the things that need to be done and not judging the goodness or badness of it all. If someone needs some extra help after we turn out the lights, I just give it to them. I don't need to mentally rehearse all the reasons why my work should be done by now. By letting go of the arguments inside my head (or sometimes out loud, with the children), I can escape the struggle and just do what's asked of me.

It doesn't mean that I wouldn't still prefer to be lying on the couch with a good book in the early evening hours. It just means that I stop thinking so much about what I can't do or don't want to do or would rather be doing. Do the kids still run wild, claiming late night hunger and bathroom urgency? Sure. But they will do so regardless, so I might as well use my energy to do what needs to be done instead of adding on the extra work of resistance.

Julia S. Aziz

Following my Own Lead

As I continued to struggle with the contractions, I began to question myself. When I lay down on the bed, doubt crept in and asked, "Shouldn't I be squatting or walking instead?" Advice from books, friendly moms, and childbirth professionals ran through my mind, but often my body didn't want to follow along. "Get in the shower," the book would say. Well, the shower in my hospital couldn't get above lukewarm even at its highest setting, and I liked my showers hot, even when I was not in relentless pain. "You should vary positions throughout labor," said the childbirth preparation class, but what if my body just liked to bend over at the waist, leaning on the bed, and anything else felt horrible? This internal confusion and debate continued between contractions. Meanwhile, my body clearly knew what it wanted to do. It wanted to lie in the bed for a while or stand and bend over at the waist, no questions asked.

Advice can be helpful, but it also can lead me astray from my own wisdom.

Upon close examination, many instructions seem to be derived from observing natural processes. Noticing that women tend to labor more easily moving around becomes the advice: "You should vary positions in labor." Advice can trigger a desire in me to do things right, to earn the gold star.

I take others' ideas as rules to follow instead of potentially useful or not-so-useful suggestions. While following these rules can sometimes be a comfort, it is not nearly as empowering as forging my own path. Just because I try to follow the rules doesn't mean they will work for me in the same way every time. It is actually more helpful to let my own natural process unfold.

Like many new moms, after my first baby was born, I became obsessed with sleep. I hungered desperately for it, and it felt entirely out of reach. I consumed books, websites, and conversations with friends like they would save my life, and they just didn't. I tried everything to get my baby to fall asleep more easily and to sleep for longer stretches, but what I ended up with was a baby who woke up four times a night and slept only the very minimum of hours. I believed that this situation reflected my lack of ability to follow directions.

My distress reached a whole new level when, at 12 months old, my baby started waking up at 4:15 a.m. every morning. Completely done sleeping and unwilling even to cuddle in bed, this crawling sweetheart was ready to begin the day. Frantic and in tears, I called an old college friend who happened to be a sleep disorder specialist and begged her to fix the situation. She had some good ideas, but I had already heard them before. None had worked for me. Still, I kept trying them, assuming that one of these tried-and-true strategies would work if I just tried harder. I couldn't just give up and do nothing, could I?

In the end, waiting it out seemed to be the only strategy that was necessary. After one excessively tiring month, my son began to sleep a little later, and we could begin our days at 6 a.m. I would have preferred much later, but it seemed to approximate a reasonable person's wake-up time. Several years later, talking to my college friend on the phone again, we remembered that earlier conversation. She was now a mother, too, and her perspective had dramatically changed. She hadn't understood before why I couldn't just implement the strategies she suggested and make it work. Now that she had a baby, she understood completely. Sometimes, nothing works, and we just have to be patient. Sometimes, we don't actually need advice, especially if that advice is just going to trigger insecurity because we can't follow it.

When baby number two came along, I didn't research the latest advice by sleep experts. I just paid attention to my baby's needs, rested when I could, and tried to worry as little as possible about the paltry number of consecutive hours I spent in dreamland. Luckily, this baby actually liked to sleep. I learned to hold him or keep him right next to my body almost constantly, and if I could manage that, he would fall asleep quite easily. When I watched my own baby and did what felt right to me instead of following a plan from a "Create the Perfect Sleeping Baby" manual, everything felt easier.

Don't get me wrong. My second baby didn't sleep better than my first because I stopped listening to experts. He slept better because he just slept better. He was a different baby with different rest needs. Trusting more in myself and my baby, instead of exerting so much effort following external guidance, made even the bad nights more tolerable.

In certain struggles, maybe the real guidance we need is permission to stop seeking advice and instead to do nothing for a while. Eventually, we will find our own way through.

Julia S. Aziz

Thinking in Circles

*In the background, a mix CD played on repeat through-
out my five hours of labor at the hospital. My husband and
I had burned this CD together and had included a track of
soothing ocean sounds between every other song. Three hours
into this repeated ocean soundtrack, I wanted the CD to be
thrown out the window or at least turned off. I was desperate
to be rid of those manufactured waves, but I could not speak
out loud to ask my husband or doula for help. Never before
had I felt such an odd separation between my mind and body.
My thoughts continued in their ranting (I wish they would
turn off that CD!), and yet I could not get the words out of
my mouth. All of my bodily functions, including speech, were
overtaken completely by the involuntary contractions of my
uterus—and my uterus was doing its job whether or not the
sounds of the ocean were soothing my mind.*

*When I could let the music be background instead of fore-
ground, my irritation would recede. In those moments, I could
breathe deeply and repeat the song I truly wanted to hear in
my mind, noticing the contractions escalate and diminish according to their own rhythm.*

**Sometimes I get stuck in a mental loop. When
my thoughts are getting me nowhere but the
same place I have been, it's time to move my attention somewhere else.**

Over-thinking, for me, has been a true impediment to parenting. Many experts seem to suggest that parenting is a science we can be trained in, rather than a relationship we need to feel our way through. The newest theories offer us specific responses to crying babies, stubborn toddlers, or fighting siblings. I get caught in this mentality, believing that if I can just keep thinking about the problems of parenting for long enough, I can solve them.

What if they aren't problems, though, but rather just the stuff of life? In that case, wouldn't it be better to just respond to my children in the moment, based on a true presence with what's actually happening? When I can step back a little from immersion in my own thoughts, I feel a slight spaciousness and more freedom to choose where I put my awareness. This doesn't mean that thoughts are the enemy. I couldn't get rid of them if I tried. Sometimes, though, it helps to place less stock in the validity of my thoughts and break myself out of those mental loops.

Right now, it's 4 a.m., and I've been awake since my son's coughing episode woke me up about an hour ago. He's okay now and has gone back to sleep, but I feel fully alert. Before I had children and in my earliest years as a parent, I engaged in serious negotiations with my mind when I would lie awake like this in the middle of the night. I'd beg, "Please go to sleep." I'd warn, "You only have three hours until you have to get up." I'd fret, "How will you be able to function at work?" I was exclusively focused on my inability to sleep. Regardless of the mental exercise, I would be awake for approximately two hours, and then I would either fall asleep or get up for the day if it was already morning.

No matter what I tried to do, those two hours felt endless, like I'd been up for days on end. I tried various sleep-inducing herbs, melatonin supplements, and prescription medications. I played with every strategy imaginable. The best one was forcing myself to scrub the shower stall tiles in the middle of the night. (The rationale was that the threat of an onerous chore would trick the mind into quickly going back to sleep. If it didn't work, I would still have a clean bathroom.) I have a good deal of willpower, but I couldn't keep trying that method for more than a couple nights.

A few years ago, I surrendered to the insomnia. I just accepted that there will be some nights I don't sleep much. Sometimes (many times), a child wakes me up, but other times it's just me, needing to go to the bathroom or waking up from a dream. Regardless of the reason, I will be up for about two hours. Accepting this pattern, I have been able to use the time to do whatever I feel like doing. Often, I will relax in bed, letting my mind wander without worrying about the time. Other nights, like this one, I get up a little and read or write.

The time is much more pleasant now. First I am asleep, and then I wake up for two hours. Then, I go back to sleep or get up for the day, just like before. The only difference is that I don't engage in mental negotiations or watch the clock anymore. If it doesn't matter what my mind is doing, if I will be awake anyway, why not just do something relaxing or enjoyable? Sure, I'm still tired the next day, but thinking too much about sleep never gave me much rest, either. If I can't be well rested, I can at least be free of my mental loops.

Julia S. Aziz

Time Awareness

As the contractions persisted, I started to wonder when labor would end. I wanted this baby out! When the nurses told me I was in transition, at eight or nine centimeters, all I could think about was how much further I would still have to go. My cervix would need to dilate a couple more centimeters, and then I would potentially have to push for hours. How much longer would I have to endure? Despite these questions, I had no sense of how much time had already passed. I had forgotten what increments of time even felt like.

Some contractions seemed to last an eternity, others mere moments. Of course, in reality, they were all probably between thirty seconds to a minute long, but in this other existence, the one of my pain-altered perspective, time was variable. When I thought only of the work still left to do, the minutes seemed to stretch on into an endless suffering. When I stopped anticipating the future and focused on just one contraction as it was happening, though, the surrender of time awareness was undeniably a relief. The pain felt almost, just almost, manageable.

When I focus on time, I am oriented only toward the predicted future. When I give time less of my attention, I experience more of the present.

I enter a new realm when I lose track of time, one that is both disorienting and expansive. I've experienced this time fluctuation in minor car accidents, when every movement unfolds in slow motion. I've also felt it in positive experiences like staying up all night talking at the beginning of a new romance. Each moment is so vibrant, and I feel very much alive. Then it's over, and time speeds up again.

Many say of parenting that the days are long but the years are short, and I agree. I have wished away too much time waiting for my baby to start eating solid food or for my toddler to outgrow the need for diapers. What about all those precious moments of life, those ones I miss when I am thinking only of the future? I don't want to need intense experiences to make me pay attention.

I thought I was aware of clock-time before having children, just with needing to be at work meetings and social engagements. I still had weekends, though, with late mornings and lazy afternoons. Then I had a baby, and time became constricted into tiny segments. Days were divided into wake-up time and breakfast time, morning time and naptime, postnap afternoon and dinnertime, bathtime and bedtime. When I started working more, I added on commute time and preschool time. Everything else needed to fit into one of these segments. Hanging out with friends with children meant either a morning playdate or a dinner that ended by 7:30 p.m.

Of course, I know many parents who manage wonderfully with a much looser schedule. I admire them, and I emulate them more as my kids get older. However, the majority of new parents I know stay and socialize for about two to three hours tops, regardless of the event. The best times I have had with friends since becoming a parent have been when our families have spent a weekend together outside of our regular routines. When we have a couple days, we stop paying so much attention to time, and the day unfolds. We laugh, tell stories, maybe build a fire, and watch the children run around and play. Eating and sleeping just happen when they happen, like they did in our pre-parenting lives. I don't need to keep an eye on the clock like I do with the morning playdate that has to end before preschool pickup. By making space in my life for these unstructured days with my children and friends, I re-experience a timelessness. I am relaxed and able to appreciate the beauty of where I am and who I am with. Usually, I also find a little more freedom when I return to my usual schedule at home. Maybe time isn't as scarce a commodity as I thought it was. Maybe there is enough time for everything, after all.

Julia S. Aziz

Losing Faith

The contractions became unbelievably powerful and close together, and they almost did me in. My husband and doula were both telling me that I was amazing and doing such a great job, but I could only shake my head no. No. Not amazing. "This sucks, this sucks," I kept thinking. I felt no fear, just pure and excruciating pain.

My body began pushing out the baby on its own accord, just as it was supposed to. I became focused on the "ring of fire," realizing with horror what this phrase really meant. In retrospect, the pushing only lasted an hour and a half, a reasonable amount of time for a first baby. To me, it was endless and inescapable. My baby was close to entering the world, but I could find no hope in that happy outcome. The medical staff joined us and cheered me on, but all I could do was shake my head no.

There will be times when I am convinced I just won't make it.

Most of us have experienced rough patches in life, where the despair, the rage, or the isolation feels bottomless. If you are reading this book today, somehow you made it through that dark period, or maybe you are making it through right now, every day. There are times in life when doubt looms like a dark shadow, and we wonder if we will be able to go on.

In my youth, I thought despondency would disappear completely from my life if only I had all the important things I wanted. It wasn't until becoming a mother that I saw things differently. Even when I had all those things I wanted, I was not immune to hopelessness.

New motherhood was different from other dark periods for me in that I could recognize the truly good things in my life. I was doing exactly what I intended to do, caring for a child I really wanted. There was actually nothing particularly "wrong" in my life, but the transition from being a self-reliant, independent adult to becoming a mother, a woman responsible for the well-being of a whole separate person in the world, was rough. I had some wonderful moments with my son and my husband, but I also had to live through some long stretches of self-doubt.

One afternoon, when I was fourteen weeks into my second pregnancy, my husband came home from work with a bad case of the flu. By the next day, my toddler son had it, too. This was no feeble flu. It was five to ten days of high fever, in addition to achiness, chills, incessant coughing, and fatigue. Despite my best hygiene efforts, within a few days I succumbed to the virus. Pregnant and acutely sick, I tried to take a minimal amount of medication, just enough to keep my fevers from spiking too high. Even though this meant prolonging and intensifying my discomfort, it was more important to me to protect my baby from unconfirmed but assumed risks. I was also taking care of my ill toddler, who happened to still be recovering from his recent broken leg. It wasn't very long before I was railing at the heavens, asking how I was supposed to be able to take care of other people while in such a state of suffering myself. I didn't believe I would make it through.

Of course, though, I did make it through. It took almost a month for all the symptoms to subside, but eventually I felt healthy and mostly capable again. The knowledge that "this too shall pass" is sometimes helpful, I think, but I also find it valuable and comforting to remember that losing faith is just part of the human experience.

Julia S. Aziz

Responding to What is Real

The doctor offered me a mirror so I could see my baby crowning, helping me to break through my despair and give the pushing process everything I had. After a lot of hard work, my baby really did come out—my whole, beautiful, six-pound-eight-ounce son. My son, it turned out, had swallowed meconium on his way out of the birth canal and was immediately whisked away to the hospital's neonatal intensive care unit for oxygen. I saw him for only a moment, across the room, but for long enough to see that he really was alive and out of my body at last. By watching the reactions of my doula, I could tell that the urgency going on all around me was important but that my baby's condition was unlikely to be life-threatening. It wasn't the initial bonding I had imagined. Still, I consented to the necessary procedures and inwardly rejoiced. My baby was here, alive, and I would know him soon.

It's not about everything going the way I want it to. It's about how I respond to what is actually happening.

In my first years of motherhood, I considered a good day to be a day when everything went smoothly—when the baby slept and ate well, when I was able to get some good exercise, and when several items could be checked off my to-do list.

Often, however, my days did not go as I hoped or expected, and then I would feel discouraged.

Now I try to evaluate my days differently by asking different questions. Instead of "Was this a day without outbursts?" I ask, "How did I deal with my child's tantrum this morning?" Instead of "How much sleep did I get?" I ask, "How did I replenish my energy after only several hours of interrupted sleep?" If I respond to whatever happens with an attitude of relative equanimity, I know it's been a good day.

This morning I got up at 6:30 a.m. after being woken five times in the night by the baby and by my sick three-year-old. I could sense the creeping thought, "This day is a wash," coming over me and consciously decided instead to try to make the best of it. Knowing I would be very tired, I purposely set fewer goals and tried to take breaks in my spare moments. Instead of focusing on what I wanted or what I wasn't getting, I focused on being gentle with myself and the children. I responded to the needs that arose, and I didn't lose my cool, despite the exhaustion. That, in my mind, is a pretty good day.

Instead of fixating on my preferences, I can look at how I receive what comes to me. It's not easy to give up what I want, but sometimes it's the simplest way to a happier existence—one where I can make myself proud no matter what happens in the world around me. I am not in charge of anything outside of myself, but what I do with what happens is all up to me.

Care of the Self

After confirming that my son was probably going to recover soon in the intensive care unit, I succumbed to total body shock. I never imagined that I would be comfortable letting my baby out of my sight right after meeting him, but I also never imagined the train wreck that was my postpartum body. It took nearly an hour for the doctors and nurses to deliver my placenta, stitch my tear, and wait for my uncooperative bladder to function so that they could release me to the recovery room. Only then was I finally able to give my attention to asking for my baby!

Motherhood does not erase the self. I need care, too.

Many of us pay lip service to self-care. "No one's happy unless Mama's happy!" is a common refrain. But in reality, moms, especially new moms, can be unbelievably selfless. In some ways, this is a beautiful, natural way of accepting the new role of mother. It is nature doing exactly what it needs to do to ensure the survival of our offspring. Unfortunately, with women, this selflessness can bleed into martyrdom. Mothers will almost compete over how much they are sacrificing for their child and ignoring their own needs. "I never exercise now! I haven't eaten for hours! I didn't even brush my teeth this morning!" Some of this neglect is absolutely understandable, especially in the first weeks with a new baby. When the self-sacrifice continues for months, or years, though, it causes serious wear and tear. If ignored for too long, sometimes a woman's body will start crying out for attention.

An urgent need for more intensive self-care has surprised me many times. After my third baby was born, I felt like I was coping relatively well with the multiple responsibilities. Then, when my baby was only a few weeks old, I developed mastitis, a breastfeeding rite of passage that includes high fever, severe pain, and a burning red breast. My midwife's recommended treatment was to both nurse and pump every hour, after following a complicated routine of hot water bottles and castor oil massage. It was not a fun day, to say the least. It was overwhelming to attend to my own body's needs while still making sure my baby, two-year-old, and five-year-old were taken care of! But if I wanted to avoid drugs (which I did, because of past reactions to antibiotics), I had to prioritize my own health.

My husband began boiling pots of water, cooking meals, and taking care of the boys solo. He winced in sympathy as I placed the steaming hot water bottles on my already burning skin. I gently but repeatedly woke the baby up to nurse more often than she wanted to, as it was the most effective way to get my milk to flow. When all my efforts didn't seem to be making a difference, I called the midwife again. She came to the house for several hours and patiently taught me the healing regimen. Everyone had to adjust a little to make room for the care I needed.

Sometimes my body speaks in a strong, loud voice to announce that I must care for myself and not put my needs second to my children's. When that happens, I am compelled to listen and respond; the longer I ignore myself the more trouble I may be in. Even better is when I listen and care for my own needs routinely, just like I routinely take care of my children's needs. For me, that means that even when life is particularly demanding, I still make time to take long walks outside, buy fresh produce at the farmer's market, and sit with a weekly meditation group. Women do not transform into bottomless vessels of giving when they have children. Mothers need their cups filled, too.

Julia S. Aziz

As I Am

One of my first thoughts after the birth was, "You don't ever have to do this again if you don't want to." It felt that bad. However, when I held my baby in my arms for the first time, everything I had been through took on new meaning. This miraculous human being was worth all the pain in the world.

The story does not end here, of course, with labor and birth complete. My body had a tremendous amount of healing to do, a process that took many weeks, if not months. This birth of my first child also jump-started the shocking reality of being a mother. I had no idea how to take care of a newborn baby. I could take courage, though, from looking back on how I had survived labor. Even though I sometimes resisted it as if it were my worst enemy, I had survived it. Maybe I didn't perfectly follow the natural birthing advice about relaxing and opening. Still, my baby was here, alive and well, and that's what mattered.

I can still be me, with all my particular flaws, and do this.

When I was in the first trimester of pregnancy with my son, I worried constantly. Having miscarried my first pregnancy, I lived in fear that I would lose this one, too. I checked for blood every time I went to the bathroom for those first few months; that's how consumed I was with my fears. "Don't worry so much. It's not good for the baby," offered well-meaning family and friends. Well, there was one more thing to worry about! Could it be that my anxiety would create an anxious, possibly late-developing child? Or worse, would it cause me to lose this baby, too? When I finally held my sweet angel in my arms, something deep within me healed. It wasn't just the longing to have a child. It was the longing to have a child while still being myself. I didn't have to be calmer, healthier, or better in some way to be allowed to have a baby. My flawed self was good enough.

We become mothers regardless of how healed we are of our own hang ups. If we waited until we were self-actualized to have children, it would be the end of the human race. So, we keep learning as we go, and we make lots of mistakes. Falling off course is part of our lifelong journey of growing and evolving, and it is part of our children's paths as well. Accepting the reality of our imperfection from the beginning makes becoming a parent a much easier transition.

We can still embrace the pure and perhaps universal motivation to be the best we can be when we become parents. Watching my innocent children grow, I want to do right by them. Becoming a mother has given me powerful incentive to change old patterns that no longer serve me. Hopefully, I can use that motivation to keep growing into the most peaceful, mature, and healthy version of myself. Perhaps even more important, through loving my children unconditionally, I can also learn how to love myself as I am.

BABY 2

Birthing Again: The Lesson of "Focus Changes Everything"

Julia S. Aziz

Remembering the Beginner's Mind

About a week before my second baby's due date, I woke up in the middle of the night to the same menstrual-like cramping that began my first labor. Excited at 3 a.m. in the morning, I woke my husband and started walking around, breathing deeply, and timing the contractions. After two high-adrenaline hours of this, I realized that the only thing that had progressed was my exhaustion. I had lost a precious night of sleep when the real sleep loss was imminent. I went back to bed, and my contractions eventually subsided until they went away completely.

When I called my midwife in the morning, I learned that false labor is commonplace with second babies. Apparently, I was not alone in assuming that I knew how labor would go just because I had been through it before.

It's best to be wary of thinking I've got it all figured out. The beginner's mind is open to all possibilities.

As a novice, I am eager to learn. Once I'm more seasoned, however, my self-assurance can make me less receptive. In parenting, many of us are open to all sorts of ideas the first time around, but when it comes to raising second children, we may think we know what to expect. Finally, we have a little experience under our belts and know a few things about children and parenting. Having that confidence is a relief and a blessing, but there is a danger in thinking we know. It gets in the way of learning, and it can blind us to the newness of each experience with each child.

My first son had an easy transition to preschool. He started going to a neighbor's home-based program when he was two years old, and except for one anomalous morning, he never batted an eye when it came time for me to say goodbye. Out in the world, he thrived on stimulation, and so school was a natural fit for him. When my second son started a small co-op preschool at the same age of two, I expected that a quick hug and kiss would do the trick, as it had with my first. I was very wrong. Weeks went by with tears and desperate "Mama, don't leave!" pleas every day that we separated. I was taken off guard, as secretly I had thought it was my parenting that allowed my first child to handle goodbyes so easily. But my second child needed something different from me, and he taught me that lesson by being the individual that he is.

Six months into the co-op program, I finally gave up. The separations hadn't gotten any easier, and my son really didn't want to be there. He needed more time and a smoother transition. Now, at four years old, he mostly runs off to play when he gets to his preschool at the Nature and Science Center. Sometimes, though, he still needs some extra love and attention. With my third child, I don't know what to expect. This, at least, I have learned.

It is disorienting to enter the unknown, but it is also dramatically life-affirming. I remind myself not to lose that aliveness just to gain some false security when I think I know the answers. I come back to the lesson of beginner's mind again and again. I watch friends have babies and learn to bite my tongue when I see them doing things that didn't work for me. Who am I to say what makes sense for their families? I watch my children experiment and try not to lead their way, even when I think I can predict the outcome. If their ideas fail, they will learn something from the experience of making a mistake. And who knows, maybe I will be surprised at what they discover.

Sometimes, as my older son loves to tell me, I am not right. What an exhilarating realization for a child! My mom and dad are not always right. It's something I need to remember about myself, too, because it opens up the possibility of learning something new and of not missing out on what is truly unique about each moment.

Julia S. Aziz

Best Laid Plans

My false labor was still fresh in my mind when I woke up with those cramping contractions again a few days later. Since it was 4 a.m., I did my best to stay in bed and ignore the discomfort for a few more hours. The morning wore on, but this time the contractions did not subside. They also did not become all that difficult to bear. I was in a state of limbo, with uncertainty prevailing.

Part of my ambivalence was that I knew today was the day my midwife was leaving town for a short weekend conference. She had told me about this conference well in advance since it would mean possibly missing my birth. I had chosen to work with her anyway, figuring my chances were still pretty good that she would be there. After all, she would only be gone for a day and a half of my whole final month of pregnancy.

It turned out that my labor was getting started just as my midwife was boarding the airplane. It was time for the backup plan. I knew her midwife partner Siobhan was intelligent and kind, though I did not know her well. That was about to change!

Good news, bad news, who knows?

I have always loved the Buddhist (or Taoist, depending on whom you ask) story about the farmer and his son:

There once was an old farmer who worked tirelessly for many years. One day, his horse ran away. When the neighbors heard about the horse, they came to visit. "What bad news!" they said, with pity in their voices.

"Good news, bad news, who knows?" the farmer answered.

The next morning, the horse came back, bringing two other wild horses along with it. "What good news!" the neighbors proclaimed.

"Good news, bad news, who knows?" said the farmer.

The following day, the farmer's oldest son tried to ride one of the wild horses. He was thrown off the horse, and his leg was broken. The neighbors visited again to offer their condolences.

"Good news, bad news, who knows?" answered the farmer.

The very next day, military officials came to the village to draft young men for the war. Because the son's leg was broken, they ignored him. The neighbors congratulated the farmer on his good fortune.

"Good news, bad news, who knows?" said the farmer.

Lessons of Labor

I think I know what's best, but do I really? I had chosen Mary, my primary midwife, for my first homebirth because she was one of the most experienced midwives in town. I liked her partner Siobhan but did not know much about her. She was younger, and so, surely, she was less experienced. It seemed, at first, to be bad news that Mary would miss my birth.

But Siobhan turned out to be a phenomenal birth attendant. She was undeniably competent and compassionate. The few bits of advice she gave me were right on target, little nuggets that I can remember to this day. I have never trusted another medical professional so much in my life, and so I am forever grateful to have worked with her.

I try to ask, "Good news, bad news, who knows?" when other plans go awry. A few weeks ago, for instance, two children and I came down with a stomach flu in the early morning hours of a weekday. It was a fierce illness, and so both my husband and I needed to take off time from work. In the sense of how sick we felt and how much juggling we had to do, it was bad news. But, that time off from work and from caretaking is what gave me the time and focus to write a book proposal for my publisher. I hadn't known when I would find the time to do the necessary research and writing, but I had wanted to get it done soon. All of a sudden, I had two days off, with no expectations aside from recovery. Once my symptoms subsided, I stayed in bed with my laptop, sipping water, sleeping, and writing. That family flu is in some way responsible for the book you are holding right now.

I never know how one thing will lead to another. The baby missed her nap. Will she be so over-tired that she cries during my work meeting, the one I have to bring her to today? It is impossible to know, even if I think I can predict the worst. Who knows? Maybe her interrupting that meeting would be a blessing in disguise. Since one thing leads to another, and I don't know the whole story yet, holding off on quick judgment is a pretty sound strategy. Whether the outcome is good or bad, it is likely to change anyway.

Anxiety and Love

By 1 p.m., labor had been consistent for hours, and I was ready for some guidance. I called Siobhan, who said she happened to be nearby and would stop by my house to check my cervix. Feeling relieved, I turned my attention to my other main concern: my son.

When I was anticipating this second birth, the number one question I had was about my son's care. He was only two years old and would likely be terrified if he had to witness his mom moaning like an animal in pain. Since I didn't want to feel pressure to be stoic in labor, I was certain that he shouldn't be present for the birth. He had never slept away from us before, and so I was somewhat apprehensive about how he would feel going to bed in an unfamiliar place. Luckily, a nearby friend had offered to take care of him, but since I didn't know how long labor would last, I wasn't sure when to let him leave.

I had been thinking about my son on and off all morning, but I hadn't actually been spending much time with him. My husband had been caring for him while I took slow walks around the neighborhood and coped with the contractions. After I got off the phone with the midwife, I took a few moments to slow down. I gave some attention to the feelings underneath the uncertainty, and I realized that below my lin-

gering anxiety was a desire to reconnect with my son before this big change happened in our lives.

So, I lay down on the bed with my son and told him how much I loved him. I told him that he would have a sleepover party at our friend's house, and when he came home he would meet his baby brother. I snuggled up close, breathing in his sweet smell as I allowed the contractions to pass through me. As we shared these precious moments, I was able to see that we both needed some togetherness before saying goodbye. Once we had reconnected in this way, I saw clearly that he would be okay, and so would I. It was time for someone else to take over responsibility for him for however long this process took.

Holding responsibility tightly can breed anxiety. By being present to the anxiety, rather than acting out of it, I am able to take care of myself and others from a naturally loving place.

The responsibility of parenthood is astonishing in its magnitude. When I become too consumed by that responsibility, anxiety takes over. These are the times I know I need to take a deep breath and find a way back into my heart. From this place of self-compassion, I am still responsible, but my actions arise out of love rather than fear or obligation.

A few weeks ago from this writing, my son suffered through high fevers for eight days straight. He would wake up in the middle of the night with temperatures of 104.9, 105.5, even 105.9. For the first five days, I was exhausted from getting up at all hours to give ibuprofen and cold baths, but I wasn't worried. I felt confident that my son had a virus and that it would pass. His fevers had always run higher than most, and his temperature had been dropping several degrees during the day (a good sign, said the nurse on-call with the doctor's office). We had been through five days of high fever with him before, and it was cold and flu season, after all. Adding on to all this logical reasoning was a gut feeling that we just needed to take good care of him and wait it out.

By the sixth day, though, I was unsure. Was this normal? Did he have some kind of awful infection that I was ignoring? Fear, doubt, and insecurity took over. I reverted to old patterns of frequent calls to the pediatric nurse and late-night internet searching. "High fever week-long young child" was not turning up any comforting results. Worse, it was taking me away from my son. While my husband brought him medicine and cool washcloths, I was busy being anxious and doubting myself. I could no longer see what was really happening in front of me. In truth, the pattern of his fevers had started to improve slightly. They just hadn't gone away yet. I couldn't see that change, though, because I was too caught up in my fear.

By the seventh night, I collapsed in tears. Releasing that pent-up tension, I could see that watching my son suffer for so long had become more than my heart could tolerate. When I allowed the tears to come, a rigidity released. I knew that it was time to seek help. I gave my son some extra cuddles in the morning and set an appointment with the pediatrician. It was unlikely she could do anything for us, but I needed the reassurance.

When we took him to the office that afternoon, the doctor found nothing unusual. By that evening, my son's fever started to wane all the way back to normal. It *was* a virus, after all.

Sometimes, when I watch my kids struggle, I get scared. But I don't want my fears about their well-being to dictate my care for them. What I really want is to deeply acknowledge their suffering and to lovingly tend to their needs. The only way I can do that is if I first attend to the fear that arises in me. When I look directly (and gently) at my anxiety, it loses its power over me. The rest unfolds as a matter of course because beneath all that fear lies an instinctive love waiting to be discovered and shared.

Opening

My husband left to drop off our son at my friend's house. Soon after, the midwife arrived and checked my cervix. After nine hours of regular labor, I was only two centimeters dilated. Some of the contractions felt pretty substantial, and this was all I had to show for it? Tired and disheartened, I was overcome with a sense of dread. "Oh yeah," I remembered. "This is what labor feels like. It hurts, and it's going to get so much worse."

I confided in Siobhan about my discouragement, and she talked to me a little about fear. I didn't think I was feeling any fear. I was not afraid to be in labor or have my baby. I just didn't enjoy physical suffering. What she was alluding to, however, was that some part of me was holding back. I hadn't surrendered to the painful process. I was shutting down in aversion, instead of welcoming my baby. I took her words to heart and said to my body, "Go ahead, I'm ready."

When I am stuck and feel like closing down, I can try opening up.

When faced with pain or adversity, I sometimes get stuck. I refuse to engage, and a part of me shuts down. That part wants to be protected, but instead of embracing my vulnerability, I guard against it. This I have learned: when I am defensive, I serve only to limit and darken my own light.

When I become more conscious of myself in that familiar dark place, I have a choice. I can open up and let some light back in.

Marriage (or any long-term committed partnership) offers plenty of opportunities for learning and re-learning how to open when we want to close. When a couple becomes parents, a whole new level of intimacy is available. The beauty of this intimacy is the shared love for the child and the adventure of becoming parents together. The challenge of this intimacy is a new era of interdependence and sacrifice. All of a sudden, the relationship isn't just about two individuals who love each other and independently interact with the world. It becomes much more about negotiation and trade-offs. The fact of the matter is that young children need constant minding and care. I can't just take a break when I want one. Every freedom I enjoy means more responsibility for my partner. This interdependence is hard to accept. The fact that we need each other and not just love each other creates vulnerability.

The easy thing to do with all this new and raw vulnerability is to close ranks around my heart. I can fight for my rights or engage in tit-for-tat transactions: "If you get two hours, I get two hours." Or, I can hide behind the never-ending minutiae of running a household to avoid conflict. After time, though, these tactics build into resentment, and the atmosphere feels stuck. Unconsciously, I close down in protectiveness, but there is another path available: opening. The path of opening is about welcoming the vulnerability of relationship and letting myself live unarmed.

My husband and I have been learning to make room in our marriage for the stuck places. Most Monday nights, after the kids go to bed, we give each other time to share whatever we have held too close to our chests. The other person just listens, without comment, and then echoes back what he or she heard. This contained process gives us a path toward clearer understanding of where each person is coming from.

We don't always find resolution. Sometimes that takes weeks or months, and some differences just stay unresolved. We often end our Monday night discussions with temporary agreements, to be continued the following week. It's really about opening our hearts to each other again, though, and not so much about the outcome of the disagreement at hand. When we end our "marriage work" time, we are usually able to move forward with a renewed sense of closeness and healing.

It's not easy breaking through an old pattern of looking out for myself first. Learning to look out for our relationship, too, takes practice. I still close down sometimes and hold back my love for the purpose of being right or getting my way, but my commitment to my husband has made me choose to open even when my ego wants to close. Again and again, I must learn to rescue myself from that stuck place and find the courage to be vulnerable.

Julia S. Aziz

Safety

So, I chose to welcome the process of labor. I was glad that the midwife offered to stick around for a little while instead of going home and waiting for me to call again. Knowing that my toddler was in capable hands elsewhere gave me palpable relief, too. These two things gave me a great sense of overall safety. I turned on a stand-up comedian show and paced around as needed. Less than an hour later, I entered hard and fast active labor.

Safety is relative.

Feeling safe in labor is probably different for you than it is for me. I know some moms who appreciated having their older children watch them give birth. Other women prefer to be alone, like an animal mother in a dark cave, and only then can their labor progress. Still others need competent professionals standing at their bedsides. For me, it was somewhat different with each labor because what I needed had changed.

During my first pregnancy, I sometimes questioned my decision to have a hospital birth instead of a homebirth. I knew I wanted to labor without pain medication. I also knew that a hospital would be a more challenging place to do so in that the staff is more accustomed to working with women who choose epidurals. But I had never given birth before, and I was somewhat besieged with fears about the safety and health of my newborn. I knew that if any emergency occurred, I wanted to be as close to medical help as possible.

None of this is unique or unusual to me. However, I happen to live in a very progressive city surrounded by very alternative-type people. At the time, most of the mothers I knew had chosen homebirths with midwives. Near the end of my pregnancy, I started having some conflicts with my obstetrician and realized that she was a lot more conservative than I had known. One of my well-meaning, well-loved friends suggested I switch caregivers and instead plan a homebirth with a midwife. I was about 34 weeks pregnant at the time, and the idea of making such a huge change at that point was positively panic-inducing. I didn't want that choice. I wanted to be able to trust in the plan I had already made. Nonetheless, the suggestion sat with me and made me question myself. Why was I not as brave as my friend? Why couldn't I be more like her, so self-assured and self-reliant? Eventually, I realized that my comfort zone differed from hers, and that was okay. At that point in my pregnancy and my life, feeling safe meant sticking with the known.

Concerns about safety increase exponentially once a woman becomes a mother. We may take risks with our own lives, but most of us are more cautious when it comes to our offspring. It doesn't help that new moms are bombarded with news and advertising that warn against a myriad of dangers that could potentially injure or kill their children. Never let your baby sleep on his tummy! Always cut your grapes into quarters! Check your home for hidden toxins! Keep your child in a car seat for as long as you possibly can! There is no end to it.

I can't tell anyone how to make choices about these things and neither can the news, friends, relatives, or parenting experts. We just have to learn what we can, decide what will help us sleep at night, and then move on. There is inherent risk in life. Put a fragile little person in my arms and make me the responsible party for his well-being, and the prospect of making so many decisions is overwhelming. The trick is to trust whatever makes me feel the most safe and to stand by my own decisions.

Julia S. Aziz

Complaining

The contractions began to draw in all my attention. I got down on my hands and knees on a futon mattress in the baby's room and went to work. My initial coping technique involved a lot of loud profanity and moaning. At some point, the assistant midwife arrived, and Siobhan filled her in on what had been happening. "She likes to cuss," she explained, which internally made me laugh. It was true. I was cussing like a sailor, with long drawn out yells of "F-ck!" through the contractions.

Complaining can be fun, but it doesn't usually serve me all that well.

Does it help to complain? Sometimes, blowing off steam is a good release of built-up pressure. Often, women's "bitching and moaning" leads to lots of laughter and camaraderie. It's a way we share our struggles and commiserate on the obstacles before us. Many a phone call or playdate has been spent bemoaning toddlers that need their apple slices not to touch their sandwiches, babies that won't sleep at night, or husbands that ignore incessant whining and continue surfing the web on their iPhones.

Then, I have to ask myself, "What does all that complaining do to my connection with the ones I am complaining about?" I have a wonderful friend whom I call when I am most passionately angry at my husband. I call her not because she will commiserate with my woes, which she can, but because she calls me on my own sh-t. She will look at the situation from my husband's perspective and help me figure out what I can do to meet him halfway. In talking to her, I can find my way back to some peace with him.

Yeah, sometimes I just want to complain. Usually, it doesn't solve the problem. In truth, painting such an ugly picture of my life and my loved ones makes me feel more disconnected from them. Complaining can be feeding the beast, giving even more fuel to indignation and frustration. It's the thought-word-deed idea. What we think about is given more power when we talk about it and even more power when we act on it. So, if I think about how unhappy I am, and then I talk about everything I don't like in my life, I just reinforce the idea that I am unhappy. When I act on that unhappiness, yelling at my kids, slamming cabinets shut, or zoning out in front of bad television, I become even unhappier. I may not be able to stop the thoughts of discontent, but I can consciously decide to redirect my attention once I notice they are there.

This is not to say that I believe in storing all my unhappiness inside or hiding my problems from friends. I would not have survived early motherhood this long without confiding in my girlfriends, and that is only a slight exaggeration. They have carried me through. Our shared honesty has lifted the isolation and consoled me with the knowledge that I am not alone. Still, even with friends, I need to keep an eye on my complaining and strive for a more balanced, grateful perspective on my life.

Just a Little Help Helps

When the cussing seemed to become counterproductive, Siobhan gently suggested that I change tactics. She told me to imagine approaching my labor like I would yoga. Her idea was to choose a mental focus while breathing slowly and deeply through the contractions, just as if I were working on a difficult yoga pose. Somehow these few words shifted me away from howling through the pain and inspired me to try a more accepting and disciplined approach.

A few choice words may be all that's needed, and they can make a big difference.

I have often found that an offhand comment spoken at just the right moment can be the trigger needed to initiate a much larger change. About a year after my second son was born, I started realizing how deep a funk I had been in for some time. I was having margaritas with a friend from graduate school, also a mom of two small children, commiserating about the hormonal and emotional challenges we had experienced. She told me that exercise had transformed her perspective, and it was like a light had been turned on for me. I needed to get moving.

I have always been a walker. Every day I walk at least a few miles. I walked before I was pregnant, while I was pregnant, and throughout the years since, but in that postpartum year after my second child was born, I wasn't getting quite the cardiovascular rush I needed to really rewire my brain. Soon after the conversation with my friend, I joined a gym, despite my self-proclaimed non-gym-person identity. Sweating through challenging aerobic exercise did wonders for my mental health. Aside from the physical health benefits, it helped me move through a lot of the frustration I was feeling. A despair I had been fighting off for a long time began to lift, and I still credit this one happy hour. Nothing my friend said was earth-shattering, but I was able to hear the wisdom of her experience at the right moment in my life. In that way, she made a truly significant difference.

Even people I don't know have made an impact on my life with just a few kind words. At least a few times a week, I push a stroller along my favorite walking trail in Austin. The child in the stroller has changed over the past eight years, but the trail has not. As I round the bend where the ducks like to swim, I often see an older musician sitting on top of a hill playing his guitar. Every time I pass him, he yells out, "Good job, Mom!" It doesn't matter what time of day or season of the year it is or that we have never had a true conversation. He sends off these well wishes to every mom he sees.

This stranger can't tell my good days from my bad, but every time I hear those words, I feel my spirits lift just a little. Random, unconditional compliments are much appreciated. We could all use a little encouragement now and then.

Gentle Focus

I consciously chose a focal point other than the pain in my body. I started spelling out my baby's name silently throughout the contractions, a funny idea that my mom had suggested weeks before. Every time a contraction started to escalate, I just breathed deeply and spelled his name slowly, over and over again. When the pain began to recede, so did my spelling game. Through practicing this gentle focus, I could follow along with the rhythm of my contractions. I wasn't working too intensely with the pain, nor was I giving up in despair. In this middle way, I struggled less, and the work of labor seemed easier than before.

Between too much effort and too little, there is a middle way of gentle focus.

When it comes to a difficult challenge, there is such a thing as too much effort. Sometimes, when I am working too hard at something, what I really need to do is sit back a little. I need to find something else to put my mind to, something easy that has no charge to it. When I let my gaze rest more gently on the task at hand, I am often surprised by new insights. Many of my best ideas have come while taking a meandering hike through the forest or a meandering journey through my thoughts in meditation. With a lighter focus, whatever I have been working on starts working itself out.

I am learning that more effort does not always lead to greater results. I can work myself harder and harder, but I may not actually accomplish more. I can only do my part in this universe, and I have to trust that all the other factors are going to do theirs. If I work too hard, I just work too hard; it doesn't mean the work is any better at all. The trick is knowing when to push harder and when to pull back.

There is no magic formula that I know of, besides cultivating and responding to a moment-to-moment intuitive awareness. I am getting worn out, I pull back. I'm feeling lazy, I push a little beyond. Like the Buddhists teach, I am at my best when I am neither too active nor too passive but somewhere in the middle. When I am focused, but not rigidly so, I find my way along this middle path.

I have always been interested in health, but my focus on it intensified when I became a mother. When my first baby started eating solid foods, I was determined to make each bite a nutritious one. His rice cereal had to be organic and only mixed with breastmilk. By the time my second baby was born, I had learned even more about nutrition and health. My second son was given no rice cereal at all because it was processed food (!), and he didn't need to be having any of that. As he was more particular about what he ate than his older brother, I had to be extra creative for him to get the same nutrition. I concocted daily smoothies filled with nutritious, local, organic greens and pancakes made out of root vegetables and beans.

The more I learned about food, the harder I worked to make our meals healthier. My sons' bodies are probably better off for all this early good nutrition, but the stress I put on myself to always have a well-designed, healthy (and edible) meal for my children did not necessarily add to our family's well-being. When I found myself turning down dinner invitations to avoid awkward conversations about food preferences and spoon-feeding my four-year-old to make sure he finished the soup I worked so hard on, it was hard to say whether "healthy" could still describe my choices.

By the time my third baby came along, I needed to find a gentler way. My children's nutrition was still important to me, but I couldn't maintain such a narrow focus on it. My daughter has had plenty of green smoothies in her short lifetime, but she doesn't get one every day. She eats a healthy array of different foods, but if she doesn't like something, I don't necessarily try to hide it in a pancake to get those particular nutrients in. When I want to experiment with new health foods, I try them myself and offer whatever I am having to my kids. If they want it, great, but if they don't, I don't push it. They still eat fresh, local, organic vegetables every day, but they also bake sugar cookies with our neighbor down the street and have days where bread and spaghetti make up the bulk of their calories.

I hope that my children learn to care for their bodies but not obsess over them. As for myself, I still vacillate between eating very well and eating poorly. I have yet to find the perfect balance, but a gentle focus on health, for both myself and my family, is my intention.

Julia S. Aziz

One Foot in Front of the Other

Because I was spelling, there was no room for negative thoughts to creep their way into my consciousness. Every time I felt pulled in that direction, I reminded myself to stay with the present experience of "just this one contraction." I didn't fight, and I didn't think about how much more time it would take for this process to end. Just this one contraction was all I needed to get through.

I only need to take one step at a time.

There is a Hebrew song we sing on the Days of Awe, the High Holy Days, which translates like this: "The entire world is a very narrow bridge. The essential thing is to have no fear at all."[1] I sang this song, in my head and sometimes out loud, throughout my pregnancy and during the birth of my first child. As I mentioned before, my earlier miscarriage made me scared I would lose that pregnancy, too. There was no way to know for sure that my baby would be okay. My doubt was somewhat relieved when I saw my son for the first time at a 20 week ultrasound, but it revisited me on and off until I held him in my arms. The song acted as an anchor for me, a

---

1 Nahman, as cited in Teutsch, D. A. (Ed.). 1994. Kol Haneshamah: Shabbat Vehagim (2nd ed.). Wyncote, PA: The Reconstructionist Press, p. 848.

reminder that the fragility I felt was real, but that all I could do was to take one step at a time across that narrow bridge.

I don't believe this Hebrew prayer is saying that we need to deny or avoid fear. I don't think we can actually control the feeling of fear arising. Instead, I believe we are meant to understand that living is as tentative and as beautiful as the experience of using a fallen tree to cross a rushing river. It is incredibly scary and yet exhilarating. If I can just focus on the task before me—the one foot in front of the other on the very narrow bridge—I can walk. The essential thing is not to focus on the fear and not even to focus on the destination. Just take one step at a time.

Even when life doesn't feel as risky, I need to remind myself to focus just on the one step in front of me. Having children so close in age means that I have had very little down time in the past decade. When I look at the whole picture of my life, it gets a little overwhelming. I can look ahead at my week and see an employee evaluation at my job, grocery shopping, my sons' piano lessons, my women's group, writing this book, doing four people's laundry, and figuring out how to work from home because two of the kids are getting sick again. That's all too much to think about. It's better to just focus on what I am doing right now, which is sitting at a coffee shop, writing. Who cares that I need to pack three lunches, make dinner, do two loads of laundry, and finish our taxes this evening? That's later.

Having three children has made this lesson of staying focused on the present more urgent and thus easier to absorb. Ironically, having too much to do compels me to surrender more often. When I am faced with more chaos than I can control on such a regular basis, I learn to just do the one thing in front of me. Perhaps this is why the patience I have had with my third baby far exceeds what I was capable of with my first two. When my daughter went through weeks of waking up every hour, I knew it would end, and so I just focused on being with her when she needed me. When weaning her took much longer than with the other two, I didn't worry about it. Since I knew she would stop nursing eventually, I just enjoyed that special bond for as long as it lasted.

So, I do my best to just be in the place I am, looking at my priorities and choosing only my next step. While I am cooking dinner, the boys chase each other with large bamboo poles, my daughter dumps beads all over the kitchen floor, the pot of beans overflows, and the smoke alarm goes off. But I can see clearly. It is time to open a window.

Julia S. Aziz

Finding the Pause

Even more liberating than my spelling technique was a new inspiration to enjoy the time between contractions. What an incredible difference it made to attend to the pause rather than the contraction, even if that pause only lasted about 30 seconds. During the contraction, I would concentrate on my slow spelling; after it, I would rest. I discovered that total rest, truly a complete break, was possible, if I just kept my mind with my body in the present moment of non-contraction. It was kind of amazing.

I still felt an intense surge of pain during each contraction, but afterward, I felt nothing. Allowing myself to relax in that nothingness was astonishing. It was a wake-up call to realize that the pain wasn't all-encompassing. In my first labor, my mind was so focused on the intensity of the pain and how soon it would come back that I couldn't enjoy or elongate the rest period. With this second labor, I could sense the build up during a contraction as well as its surrender. I saw the truth that the slow crescendo of pain really does release.

Even in times of great effort, there are periods of rest. I can let the pauses be my foreground.

There is a fine distinction between waiting and pausing, but it is a good one. When I am waiting, I am holding my breath, figuratively if not literally, until the next (good or bad) thing happens. When I pause, I am not awaiting any future; I am just resting. It's lovely.

Sometimes, with a family of five, it feels like there is always something off. There is always someone sick, upset, not sleeping well, or arguing. It is easy to get dragged down under the barrage of troubles and each individual's reaction to them all. But then, there are those moments—we all have them—of relative peace. My sons might be playing outside in the tree fort while I am cooking dinner, and my husband is carrying the baby while washing dishes with a free hand. It's all okay for the moment. We're doing just fine.

Even when I had just one baby, it wasn't always easy to find the pause. My baby's naps were often short as his pattern was to sleep for just 20 minutes, an hour if it was a lucky day. I would begin tensing up when 18 minutes had passed, just waiting for that wake-up cry. I would be thinking, "It's not enough, not enough time." But there were two minutes left, maybe even more, and if I consciously let go, I could use that little time to do some deep breathing. Or stretching. Or whatever was restful for me.

These are the pauses in-between, the times when everything is settled for a minute. Instead of waiting for the next task or the next crisis, I let out a big exhale. I take what rest I can get, no matter how short-lived. Sometimes, a five-minute catnap restores my energy even better than if I had slept for an hour. The more I cultivate this attitude of enjoying the pauses that arise naturally, the more these little pauses genuinely give me the respite I need.

Less Can Be More

There were no more inspections of my cervix at this home-birth. Aside from that initial time when the midwife arrived and found my dilation to be only two centimeters, she never checked me again. When I labored in the hospital with my first baby, the nurses had checked my cervix at least three or four times. Certainly, they had needed to check me before giving their approval on my pushing the baby out. When my body started pushing in this second labor, I wondered aloud if the midwife would need to give me the O.K. to move on to this final stage. To my surprise, she told me to just allow the pushing to happen, without making sure I was fully dilated. Now, this makes total sense to me, as obviously my body would start pushing when there was room for the baby to come out. At the time, however, I was quite intrigued by how little external information the midwife wanted and how different her approach was from the scientific, hospital-based method. I observed it all in my mind, this newness of just trusting my body without all the measurements and external validation.

Less information is often more useful to me.

There are many instances in pregnancy when we are faced with the question of how much information to seek out or take in. There are blood tests, for instance, that are offered near the end of the first trimester. Some women automatically assent to being tested for any fetal abnormalities that are detectable, while others decline the opportunity. There are so many tests these days, so many monitoring devices, that we may just go along and think more is better when it comes to information.

For some women, all this information is a huge comfort. The more they know, the safer they feel. For others, more information is actually more stress-producing. I turned down the blood tests that were available when I was pregnant, mainly because I didn't want to know a statistic about my chances of something. At the time, those blood tests could only determine a probability of having a child with chromosomal abnormalities, and that particular information wouldn't actually tell me anything definitive about my own baby. Also, I knew this kind of information could produce more stress if I worried about something that I didn't have to actually deal with yet.

But that's just me. I have learned that I am someone who actually does best with less information. I no longer read parenting books aside from personal memoir types. I employ my best self-discipline to not research health concerns by scouring the internet. And I don't use a thermometer to take my kids' temperatures unless they feel unusually hot. It's not because I want to ignore their symptoms but because I have learned that I can tell through visual observation and touch when they are truly sick. I can tailor their care to that knowing, rather than to a number.

When I know an exact temperature, it is useful for telling the doctor (when a doctor is needed). Aside from that, the thermometer just keeps me focused on the numbers rather than on my sick child's behavior and symptoms. I am not advocating that parents throw away their thermometers. I wouldn't do that; I even take one with me when we travel. When faced with a desperately sick child in an unfamiliar place, I want all the information I can get. But even though mine may be the minority perspective on this, I do know what is true for me: the less external information I can get by with, the less distracted I am from my own perceptions and intuitions. And over time, the more I seek out internally sourced information, the more reliable my discernment becomes.

Julia S. Aziz

Trust

We were all a little surprised that the baby didn't come out in just a push or two, since second labors often end in easy pushing. After about thirty minutes, my baby's head had emerged, but the midwife could see that his shoulder was stuck. "Julia, you need to push this baby out right now," she told me, even though there was no contraction to help him along.

Much later, I watched the video of my son's entrance to the world and was astonished at how blue his face looked in these moments of limbo. His head was suspended outside of me while his body was stuck inside. I could see how truly urgent the situation had been, and it looked pretty scary. At the time, however, I felt no fear or doubt, just determined focus. I trusted that my midwife knew what she was doing and that if she was giving me a directive, I was capable of following it.

Mustering all my strength and will, I did as I was told. The midwife assisted me by shifting the baby's shoulder, and that was all it took. He came all the way out, and within moments, he was in my arms. At 4 p.m., just two and a half hours after the midwife had arrived, my baby was born.

When I am willing to trust, I am surprised by what is possible.

Sometimes I am faced with a challenge so unfamiliar and daunting, I cannot lead my own way through it. When I can't see but still have to leap, all that's left to do is trust. Trust is the antidote to self-doubt, one that does not rely on a false bravado but instead authentically and courageously embraces the unknown. What does it mean to trust, and how do I become more trusting? When I look deeply into the trajectory of my life, I see that this is one of my guiding questions. I am always being taught the lesson of trust; as each unfamiliar situation comes my way, I receive yet another opportunity to learn. What I know so far is this: when I approach life's uncertainty with a willingness to not know the answers, more is possible than I could ever dream of.

Before having children, I loved to explore new places. My husband and I had each traveled solo internationally in our twenties, and though we became more settled into work and home when we married, we still escaped on frequent roadtrips to the ocean. Once we became parents, though, our travels became much tamer. New adventures felt too complicated with all the extra planning, the heavy baby paraphernalia, and the mercurial temperament of our new traveling companion. On top of the effort involved, self-doubt made me reluctant to journey far. I was apprehensive about sleep, privacy, food, health emergencies, and anything else that would need to be handled differently if we were far from home. Basically, I lacked the confidence to parent without the comfort of our routines. So, for the first few years of parenthood, we visited my mom in Massachusetts once a year, but we didn't do much exploring outside of the known.

After such an extended time developing some domesticity and staying close to home, my free-spirited side longed to fly. With three children, travel would clearly be even more challenging, but my wanderlust had returned. I didn't want to hide behind my fears anymore. I realized that there would always be good excuses to live a more narrow life with children, but it was time to dream again and to include our children in those dreams.

So, last summer, our family took a five-week road trip across seven states. It was a somewhat epic adventure, as we alternated between camping in national parks, crashing with family and friends, and attending two weddings along the way. Before we left, I had no idea how it would go. I was still nursing, and the baby was still in diapers. Since the five of us would have to sleep in one room or tent together for four out of the five weeks, sleep (and privacy) would be at a bare minimum. How would we even fit all our camping gear in the car, let alone live out of it for over a month?

Though it was uncharted territory, we headed down the road. We had a tire blow out, various bouts of illness, and more than a few sleepless nights, but we also had hours of running up and down sand dunes and hiding under big redwood trees. As we drove back to Texas on our last leg of the trip, I looked back at my kids in their car seats and saw something unprecedented. My oldest son was reading to my youngest, and my daughter was napping (the first car nap in five weeks!). We had hit our roadtrip groove. I was struck by the possibility that we could live a more adventurous life than the one we had been living. I didn't need to live my life smaller just because I was a parent.

Lately I have been dreaming of leading retreats and living closer to nature somewhere in northern California. I am often told that it is too expensive to live there, especially with a family of five. But people do it. Why not us? Trusting more deeply, I am excited not to know what's next.

Julia S. Aziz

The New Normal

My baby had arrived healthy and whole. I spent the rest of the afternoon recovering and admiring my son in all his perfect newness. We happily greeted my older son in the morning, as he came home and shyly studied his new brother. Suddenly, we were no longer a family of three, but a family of four. It was a whole new world, and we would need to find our way around it. We had no idea how things might change, but we were grateful to be at the start of something new together.

The new normal will not be the old normal, but there will be a new normal eventually. The time between the two is temporary, and it is beautiful in its own way.

Recently I talked to a new mom about how she was anxiously anticipating the time when she would have to take care of her newborn daughter alone. Her mother was visiting her in the first weeks after the birth, and because of this, she wasn't doing any of the household chores like cooking, cleaning, or running errands. She was just nursing the baby and recovering. She was doing pretty well with these two tasks, but she was scared of what it would be like when she had to take on all the usual obligations again. I told her that when she was alone and forced to cope on her own, she would. She would figure it all out in her own time. These days of learning to be a mother, and of her mother learning to be a grandmother, would soon end.

The transition from having no children to having a child is, by every measure, a huge one. Life is turned on its head. A couple's division of labor in the household gets renegotiated, friendships are altered, work schedules shift, sleeping arrangements change, and everyone becomes a little disoriented. A new, vulnerable member of the family must be accommodated into the life pattern, and what used to work well can become impossible. Eventually, a new order is established, and everyone generally knows where they fit in again. It's that time in-between that is so precious because when everything is up in the air, anything can happen. All possibilities are open. While it is unsettling not to know how to handle everything, not knowing also has a certain beauty. Many new parents experience something like a honeymoon in this in-between period, one of great gratitude, laughter, tears, and a true vulnerability that brings everyone closer. Between the old normal and the new normal routines, there is connection and learning.

While having a second baby might not be as dramatic a transition as having a first baby, it does still disrupt an established pattern. When my second baby was born, I spent a month in bed with him. That may be a slight exaggeration, but only slight. As a teacher, my husband had the summer off, and so he was able to take care of our toddler while I recuperated and bonded with the baby. Our toddler had to adjust to this shift in his primary caretaker, and my husband and I had to adjust as well. The situation was temporary, as the school year would start up again in a few weeks, but for that time in between, I was given this gift of fully devoting myself to my new baby and to regaining enough strength and energy to take over when my husband went back to work.

Lessons of Labor

Spending so much solo time together, our older son became more attached to his father than before. The baby and I, too, found an easy and blissful connection to each other. I learned how to nurse him according to his own unique pattern of snacking and sleeping, and he learned how to squirm over and snuggle up to the warmth of my body. While I missed spending more time with my toddler, I also loved when he would visit us and interact with his newborn brother, pretending to nurse his stuffed animals and carrying them around in a sling. We were all learning something new, together.

When my husband went back to work, everything shifted again, and I had to work my way through the learning curve of caring for a newborn and a two-year-old together. Eventually though, a new homeostasis was found. If I can remember and trust that life always finds its way back to balance, I can more easily enjoy those temporary times in between.

Julia S. Aziz

BABY 3

Birthing One Last Time:
The Lesson of
"Try Doing It the Easy Way"

Julia S. Aziz

Whatever Works

Some mild cramping contractions woke me up at 5 a.m. one morning a few days before my third baby's due date. Even though I was clearly beginning labor, I told my husband to go to work. He would only be able to take a limited number of days off from teaching. I knew from experience that each one of those days would be precious once the baby came, especially since we would soon have three to care for. Was this a prudent course of action, for him to leave me alone with the boys while in labor? The imagined voices of family and friends answered in unison: "No!" It may not have been a plan others would choose, but still, it felt okay to me.

I need to do what works for me, not someone else.

Without even intending to, I often look to other women to answer questions in my own life. I don't think this habit is unique to me. It seems to go back to a time when my girlfriends and I would consult each other before getting dressed for middle school. So now, as an adult, if my friend is content staying home full-time with her kids, shouldn't I be, too? Answer: only if I genuinely am content. There is no "should" about it. If my friend hires a babysitter for date nights every week, shouldn't my husband and I be doing that? Answer: well, no, because we can't afford it, and she can.

Why do I bother asking these questions? I think it is because I want to know that I am acceptable, that I am worthy, and that it's really okay to be who I am and live how I live. No one else can give me that validation, though. I need to make my own choices. I can't tell you what to do any more than you can tell me. We are different people, with completely different histories, relationships, incomes, and temperaments. We can inspire each other, but we can't always answer each other's questions. All I can do is be as true to myself as possible, and let that be enough.

When my kids were one, four, and six, we drove a few hours to a friend's weekend-long wedding. Some of our closest friends attended as well. The other four families with children decided to stay together in a big cabin dorm, which sounded like a lot of fun. They were looking forward to hanging out at night when all the kids went to sleep, and they wanted us to join them.

At the time, I had trouble nursing with lots of people around, not for modesty's sake but because my skin would tear if the baby was distracted and pulled this way and that. Also, our one-year-old was still pretty young, and sleep was still a big priority (for us parents, not so much for her). So, our family chose to stay in a screened-in cabin shelter that was a long walk or short drive away from our friends. I missed being able to socialize, and I had to put aside some uneasiness about potentially being judged as inflexible or unfriendly. Still, we had to do what worked for our family. In doing so, I was reminded of how accepting our friends are and of how my self-consciousness stems mostly from my own judgments and projections. In the end, it's okay just to do what works for me.

The Big Picture

So, I kissed my husband goodbye. Thus began one of the strangest, most surreal days I have ever experienced.

My boys were then five and two years old, and both were awake and needing assistance by 6:30 a.m. I got them dressed, helped them brush their teeth, and made breakfast while they vacillated between tired crying and begrudging cooperation. Meanwhile, my body was having contractions every five to ten minutes. On top of all that, my mind, while half-attentive to the boys' needs, was racing with decision-making questions: should I drive my oldest to preschool? Is it safe to drive while in labor? What if I am okay on the way there but then in hard labor on the way back? How will my son get home if labor progresses while he is at school for the next four hours?

In addition to the morning routine, the contractions, and the planning questions, I was enjoying a meta-awareness of the whole situation. It was truly bizarre to be entering one of the most life-altering events possible in a human life while still frying up some eggs, wiping bottoms, redirecting tantrums, and enduring regular intervals of pain. With all these disparate experiences at once, I felt like I had entered a somewhat altered consciousness. I wrote in my journal that morning: "Life is hilarious, crazy, beautiful, and absolutely unknown."

If I step back, I can see the big picture.

In labor, oxytocin invited me to enter a grander consciousness than my usual frame of mind. Without such a surge of hormones, though, I sometimes struggle to see the big picture. When there are too many things going on at once, I can't always see clearly what my life is all about. When I am the only responsible adult around, I cannot always escape the chaos to find perspective.

My first year with two small children was the most challenging of my early motherhood years. My active two-year-old loved to climb and explore anything and everything he could. When I would sit down to nurse the baby, he would take the opportunity to sneak up on the kitchen counter and remove all the dishes. To ensure his safety and my sanity, I needed to take him outside a lot. I would nurse the baby in a sling while guiding my toddler up the trees at the park and chatting with the neighborhood moms. It may have looked somewhat manageable on the outside, but internally, the lack of rest, the hormones, and the constant multitasking were wearing me down.

About mid-year, I started receiving clear signs from my body that something needed to change. Minor, commonplace events were triggering excessive levels of stress. My son would be attempting to escape out the side door by dismantling the child safety lock while I was getting dressed and consoling the crying baby. Then, suddenly, I would be breathing fast and shallow, with locked jaw and racing heart. After some time, the symptoms would disappear, but I would be shaken to the core. It felt like the chaos around me was invading my nervous system.

It took some time, a renewed commitment to my meditation practice, and some long talks with my former therapy colleagues, but I learned some tools to prevent the panic. I became aware of how and when the outside stimulation began pervading my body. When I felt the rush of stress coming on, I would stop what I was doing and breathe deeply. Since I was alone with the children, I didn't have the luxury of stepping away from the situation physically, but once I was calm, I could step away in my mind.

Seeing the bigger picture was just what I needed. From a more expansive awareness, I could see that my children and I were often reacting to each other in a swirl of activity and emotion. We were all still learning and doing our best, bumbling along but still moving in a somewhat forward direction. From the right point of view, my life with kids was more a comedy than a suspenseful thriller.

Chaos, at least the kind I experience in family life, seems to have an energy all its own, and sometimes the broader view completely eludes me. When I do find a way to step back and see the big picture, I am often entertained by the show.

Julia S. Aziz

The Unforeseeable Future

My sons and I went about our usual morning routine, the main difference being that I was in labor. One of the most poignant moments of that morning still shines in my memory, clear as day. My older son came over to me as I was bending over for a contraction and asked, "What are we going to do today?" I answered, "I have absolutely no idea." To which he responded, "Wow! That's cool!"

I never know what's going to happen next. Sometimes this truth is frightening, and sometimes it's liberating. Either way, like my son said, "Wow! That's cool!"

I found this interchange with my son to be funny and telling. You see, I always have a plan, and my oldest child knows this better than anyone. Even on our more relaxed, spontaneous days, I have some ideas about what to do. Rarely do I admit to my children how little I truly know about what's going to happen, as I often operate under the assumption that children like to know what to expect. In the big picture, though, every day is unpredictable. Why not teach by example how to embrace the unknown?

Days on end caring for small children can sometimes be tedious and isolating, not to mention the guilt that arises for feeling that way. It can seem like *Groundhog Day*; over and over again, same in, same out. To think like this is to invite depression, but to wake up each morning, wondering what this particular day will bring, remembering that anything could happen, is to live with hope and wonder. It's much easier said than done, but even if I can catch a glimpse of this way of seeing a few times a day, even once a week, I open my eyes to the mystery of living.

When an ultrasound showed that I was going to have a second boy, I wondered if I would be able to love him the way I loved my first. I felt so enamored with my son, so wholly devoted. In some secret place, I believed that this love I felt was singular and only for him. How could I ever feel that way about another little boy? I thought I would probably learn to love my second child but assumed it might take some time to get to know him.

I was entirely wrong. From the moment the midwife handed my second baby to me directly after his birth, I was a goner. It was as if I had always known him, and we had finally come back together again. Because he was born without complication, he wasn't whisked away from me like my first had been. I wasn't distracted by the shock of labor or the concern for my baby's health. I just got to hold my son. In those first moments, I knew that I had never needed to worry about not loving him enough. He was my love, right away and forever.

Wow, that's cool! I really had not believed it was possible. Surely, other moms had told me it would be this way, but I couldn't understand it then. How incredible it was that I could still love my first child so completely, and then that love would expand even larger to include his brother! When I see just how unpredictable this life is, just how much I can't foresee, I'm in awe.

Making Choices

It was time to make a decision. Should I go about my day as usual? Should I stop everything and admit that labor had begun and that today was the day? There was no clear answer, not from my body, my midwife, or my friends. I just had to make a choice.

So, I decided to take my son to preschool. I figured that I could only make a choice based on the information that I currently had, which was that the contractions were mild. I called my husband to let him know what was happening, and then we were on our way.

I can only choose based on what I know now. I can consider my options, but at some point, I just have to make a decision.

I remember packing the car for my first non-pediatrician-centered outing with my first baby. I was overwhelmed with not knowing what I might need while we were out. How many diapers would be necessary? Should I carry him around in his infant car seat or in a sling? Where would I nurse him if he got hungry? To my novice and emotional mama brain, these simple challenges were almost insurmountable. I felt pride and a slightly panicked euphoria when we successfully finished our first small errand. Over time, I learned what worked for me, and now I don't even bother bringing a diaper bag on my outings with the baby. I just take my chances and keep a couple diapers in the car for emergencies. I still don't know what I will need every time I leave the house, but I know what I will maybe need. That guess is good enough.

Decisions are easier to make when I don't wait for absolute certainty to arrive. Much to the surprise of our friends and family, my husband and I purposefully chose to have a third child. Their surprise was well-founded. We both can be somewhat introverted people who enjoy healthy doses of solitude and independence. Three children would certainly make alone time harder to come by. Besides, there were many other reasons not to have more children after our second baby was born. Finances would obviously become even tighter than they already were. I was over 35 and had been lucky to have two healthy children. Why risk it? The con list was endless, and the pro list had really just one item: it felt like one of our family members had not yet arrived. It was more of an intuitive feeling than a rational argument.

We spent months considering the various factors, but this underlying intuition didn't care. In the summer of 2010, it was time. There was no real reason why it was time, except to say that we were done thinking about it. No matter how much we contemplated the decision, the desire wasn't going anywhere. I realized that it wouldn't go away until either I had a baby or until I was past the age of when pregnancy could be an option. We had not figured out a sound financial plan or answered any of the other doubts. We just allowed and welcomed a new family member because there was love left to give. We have never regretted the decision, even once, because our daughter is such a delight. She brings joy to all the members of our family. Whatever extra work it takes to have three children is outweighed by the overwhelmingly beautiful spirit she brings to us all.

Lessons of Labor

It seems to me that parenting involves an endless series of decisions I make in the face of very little clarity about the best course of action. I gather what information I can, and then I just have to act. Sometimes, I will get the chance to choose again and change directions, and sometimes I won't. But life keeps moving on, and so do I.

Julia S. Aziz

Productive Distraction

As per my usual day, after dropping off my older son at preschool, I took my younger son for a stroller walk on a nearby trail. I asked a friend to push the stroller up the hills for me. I was, of course, still having contractions and figured that exerting myself too much was probably unwise. Still, walking on that trail every day was one of my greatest joys. Since I knew I'd have to miss it for a while in my postpartum recovery, I decided that walking with a friend would be a nice distraction from the contractions. As a bonus, maybe the movement would even get my labor going.

Productive distraction can be a very good thing.

During my first pregnancy and labor, I could not understand the advice given to me by so many books and childbirth educators: "Do something distracting in early labor." They suggested watching a movie, going out to dinner, and undertaking all sorts of everyday activities. I was so consumed by the largeness of what was happening to me (I am really having a baby now!) that these kinds of distractions couldn't draw in a fraction of my attention. I am also someone who likes to face life head-on. Instead of avoiding the pain through distraction, I thought I should dive directly into it. My plan was to meditate on it and through it.

In this third labor, however, I found myself naturally distracted. There was no need to come up with things to do, no time for movies or dinners out at restaurants. I had to take care of a preschooler and a toddler. Those responsibilities made a huge difference in my pain awareness and overall sense of calm. I couldn't feel pain as strongly when my mind was occupied.

Writing this book has been a gratifying distraction from the constant demands of having a now eight-month-old, three-year-old, and five-year-old. As I write, the baby is loudly resisting her nap in her crib, and my three-year-old is littering the entire house with streamers, tape, and cotton balls. If I were to focus exclusively on these two experiences right now, I would feel frustration and that underlying lack of purpose that stay-at-home moms seem particularly prone to. Instead, I am distracted by a creative endeavor that requires at least a third of my brain (the other two-thirds being occupied by the children). Being creatively distracted helps me get through the day in a much better mood. It even helps me parent with more patience because I am less involved in trying to control the chaos around me.

I will admit, writing while mostly ignoring my children is pretty slacker mom of me. Many women would be appalled at my inattentiveness, perhaps rightly so. However, what I am learning at this moment in my life is that I need to do whatever it takes to keep myself in balance. My feeling balanced may be the most essential ingredient to a healthy, happy home.

In that difficult postpartum year after my second son was born, I was depressed and depleted, plagued by nonstop thoughts of how badly my days were going and how I was failing my kids in too many ways. The productive distraction that works for me now will certainly not work for everyone, but I do know that moving my attention away from self-criticism and toward something purposeful has helped me pull through.

Throughout the past few years, I have taken on small independent projects. I've edited a quarterly journal, led some workshops, designed a website, and facilitated a monthly group. I have pursued these activities in addition to caring for my children full-time and working part-time. Even though it may sound like I'm pulled in many different directions, in truth, the vast majority of my hours have been spent at home caring for the needs of small children. While I love my children dearly and find a deep sense of fulfillment in being their mom, my life purpose is not wholly defined by motherhood. I know that at some point soon, my children will need me less, and I will have more time to pursue other interests. For now, my smaller-scale projects serve as an anchor to my personal dreams and a productive distraction from my 24-7 responsibilities at home.

Julia S. Aziz

Go Easy

After walking a three-mile loop, I returned home with my younger son, my soon-to-be middle child. I was tired from waking up so early that morning, and the consistent contractions were already beginning to wear me down. I asked my husband to leave work to pick up our oldest son from preschool, and I rested on the couch while my younger son napped. At around 4 p.m., I called my midwife again to consult. She told me that third labors often move slowly at first and then can stop and start up again later. She had seen this kind of pattern sometimes last for days or even a week! Realizing that a long process was a possibility, I asked for her advice on how to sleep through the contractions at night and told her I would check in again if anything changed.

When dinnertime approached, my husband and I took the kids to Central Market, a local restaurant/grocery store. While my family ate pizza, I slowly walked the grocery aisles in a labor-induced stupor. I had to stop every five minutes or so to let a contraction pass. Some were easy; some were hard. I eventually made it to the cashier to purchase the herbal remedy my midwife had recommended. When we got home, we set the boys up in the playroom with nonstop movies while my husband and I settled in on the couch and watched a silly romantic comedy. Since screen time in our house is normally restricted to a certain hour in the afternoon, the boys were delighted. It was the easiest way for everyone to co-exist happily.

The world is a better place when I go easy on myself, my kids, and my partner. Lowering my standards helps me get through.

Breathing in, breathing out. Sometimes the best course of action is just to breathe and do what's easiest. A typical morning for me might include watching one child vomit all over the carpet while a baby cries in a leaky diaper and another child tantrums about wanting me to cut out some construction paper shapes. Not all of my time is like that, but much of it really is. The stricter my agenda in these situations, the more my frustration escalates. These are the times I need to remember to go easy.

I once learned a song at a women's healing circle:

> I will be gentle with myself.
> I will love myself.
> I am a child of the universe,
> Being creative at each moment.

That pretty much sums up what I mean by going easy. I could also substitute "myself" with any one of the members of my family:

> I will be gentle with my husband.
> I will love my husband.
> He is a child of the universe,
> Being creative at each moment.

It can be challenging to see the part of each person that is childlike and pure. Even my babies, so blameless in their innocence, can exhibit such difficult behavior sometimes that

I lose sight of how simple things can be when I just go easy. What does this mean? It means I let the baby sleep wherever we both sleep the best, whether that's together in bed or in separate rooms. It means when my husband forgets to put away the orange juice, the leftover spaghetti, and the open bottle of vitamins, I just put them away and move on. It means when my three-year-old wants me to stay a few more minutes at preschool even though I am rushing to my next appointment, I take a deep breath and give him the extra attention and hugs. It especially means that I go to bed early when I need to, eat nutritious but simple meals, and do anything that makes my life easier and more nurturing.

Going easy points directly at lowering standards. If having three children has taught me anything, it has been to lower my standards. I gave everything I had to the continual assessment and service of my first baby's needs. By the third, I now give everything I have to the whole family picture. That means not everyone is as closely monitored. I often need to let go of a strict adherence to regular mealtimes or a desire for a somewhat presentable house. When I really let go, with no internal or external whining about it, it's all just fine. We're all okay, we love each other, we're healthy, and we have everything we need.

When my boys were both under the age of three, my husband had to drive seven hours to his hometown to be with his father as he was dying. Without prior warning, I was given the task of getting myself and the children down to Brownsville for the funeral within a few days. I had barely been hanging on as it was, and now the stakes were even higher. I won't say I handled this period with unshakable grace, but I did figure out how to operate in survival mode. We ate take-out every night, did away with baths, watched extra videos, and played with friends while packing. Any extra energy I could find was needed for being emotionally present to my grieving husband.

Sometimes, I cope better when the situation is more difficult. This is because I allow myself to lower my standards in a crisis. But I don't need for life to be so precarious in order to access the wisdom of this lesson. I can go easy just because I feel like it. I can be gentle with myself and my family anytime perfectionism creeps in. Letting go of ideal standards takes some practice, especially for someone like me, but it makes our family life a lot more enjoyable.

Real Acceptance Brings on Real Change

The kids finally went to sleep around 9 p.m. I continued to hang out with my husband, still experiencing contractions every five minutes until around 10 p.m. when I decided to go to bed. By this time, I had made a full mental shift. I was no longer expecting my baby to arrive soon. My new approach was just to live with the contractions and try to get some rest.

Through some tired confusion in getting ready to sleep, I miscalculated the proportions of the herbal concoction meant to calm my contractions for the night. Instead of 30 drops of the tincture, I had prepared 30 droppers-full of it. After realizing my mistake, I called the midwife to see what I should do about it. As we spoke, she remarked that I had twice stopped talking in order to breathe through the contractions. Since I sounded a little different than before, she asked if I wanted her to come over. In talking to her, I realized that maybe labor was finally progressing now that the day was over, the kids were asleep, and I had given myself permission to relax.

When I desire change, I sometimes get caught up in wanting what I do not have. Once I truly accept the way things are, they seem to shift on their own.

I have often marveled at how life offers much of what I wish for, but not right away—not when I am wishing for it. Sometimes when I am dissatisfied with a situation, I day-dream about new beginnings elsewhere. With time, whatever was bothering me often works itself out, or it stays the same, but I find a way to be happier anyway. After I've reached a place of acceptance, some of those daydreams may suddenly become real possibilities. Then, I have to decide what to do because change does not happen on my timeline, and I may no longer want those things I used to wish for!

For a long time, I identified myself as a stay-at-home mom who worked, rather than a working mom. I used this distinction mainly to convey that I was home during all the regular working hours of the week. Some of my work could be done from home, and when I did need to be gone, my husband was always there to take care of the kids. It didn't make much of a difference financially if I stuck with this set-up or worked full-time while paying for full-time childcare. After a few years of this arrangement, however, I began to crave a "real" job again, one that would get me out of my yoga pants and force me to have adult conversations that had nothing to do with parenting. Though I still wanted to be with my kids and enjoyed the flexibility of my days, I felt pulled toward contributing more to the community and re-establishing some kind of professional identity.

Somehow, as much as I desired worldly work, I couldn't find the time or the drive to seek out another job. After five years, I was finally starting to get the hang of the stay-at-home mom gig. So, instead of job searching on Craigslist, I started committing to 30-day challenges. Each month, I chose a different personal goal to focus on. I accepted that I would stay home for at least another year, while my last baby was still so young, and I would pour my need for more purpose into these challenges. In fact, writing every day on this book was my first 30-day challenge. With this renewed intention and ambition, I started to feel really good about my life and my choice to be a stay-at-home mom. Then, a month after I had truly embraced this decision, I ran into a former mentor in the parking lot of our neighborhood grocery store. She mentioned that there was an open position where she worked. Within two weeks, a job offer was in my hands.

Since change seems to come when I have stopped needing it, I am often unprepared when it arrives. Ironically, having finally embraced where I am at, I am called to welcome the new.

Julia S. Aziz

Attitude

Still feeling like I could manage on my own, I told the midwife that I would call her back in an hour if I needed her. Otherwise, I would just continue on my own. Since there had been stronger contractions throughout the day that had never developed into something more, I still felt some ambiguity about what was happening.

I decided to call my friend Louise, who agreed to sleep at our house in case the boys needed anything while I was in labor. Still relaxed about it, I told her to come whenever she was ready, no rush.

I started to move around the house, finding blankets and pillows for our guest. I asked my husband to start preparing the homebirth supplies, just in case. I figured it couldn't hurt to have it all ready. As we were moving about, I started losing focus and became unable to finish my sentences coherently. Because I had been functioning so well, figuring out where to put things and handling the contractions on my own without complaint, neither my husband nor I realized how far my labor had progressed.

When I have a relaxed attitude, I am less aware of discomfort.

Recently, my boys asked me ahead of time what I would like for my birthday. I told them that the best gift they could give me would be a day of no fighting and no complaining, just a lovely day of getting along. Knowing I can't control their behavior, I wasn't expecting much, but I thought it was worth answering their question truthfully.

On the morning of my birthday, my younger son showered me and my bed with construction paper hearts and about ten cards containing various messages of love. I snuggled him close and thanked him profusely, curiously watching my older son who had come in empty-handed. I didn't say anything and didn't mind the lack of gifts, but I was surprised since he had always been big on birthday presents. Later that day, we all went for a hike in the woods. My younger son started complaining about being tired and hungry while my two-year-old daughter cried to be picked up. Up ahead, my older son hiked quietly. I caught up to him and remarked on how nice it was that he was enjoying our hike. "I'm complaining, but only in my head," he said. "Because it's your birthday, I'm trying to get along." Surprised and touched, I hugged him and thanked him for listening to my birthday wishes. Then, I told him that not complaining on the outside was just Step One. Step Two would be to not listen to the complaining in his head. I told him that it was unlikely he could stop the thoughts of discontent in there, but he could give them less attention. Maybe he could pay more attention to the trees, the rocks, and the flowers in bloom. Who knows? By entering a more relaxed frame of mind, he might end up feeling less of the discomfort that he had been internally complaining about.

You never really know what a child (or an adult, for that matter) picks up from you. Just last night, after doing some rather uninteresting errands together, my son told me he had been practicing Steps One and Two. It took me a moment to recognize that he was referring to our earlier discussion. But it was true. He was giving less power to negative thoughts and was instead embracing a more relaxed mindset. Just like I, too, am learning how an easier-going attitude helps me ignore mild discomfort. Not only do I experience less suffering, but also I get to notice the good stuff happening, like being able to learn something new with my child.

Julia S. Aziz

Watch and Learn

At some point, I noticed that every time a contraction came on, I was instinctively getting down on the ground. I wasn't in unbearable pain, and yet my body was acting similarly to how it did when I was quite far along in the labor process with my other two babies. It dawned on me that active labor had probably begun.

My husband called the midwife to ask her to come over and continued his project of setting up the birthing area. I assumed the contractions would become a lot more difficult to bear, but in the meantime, I was happily moving along. Following an impulse for warmth and water, I moved toward the shower. Though I didn't know how dilated or effaced my cervix was, my body knew just what it needed.

I can learn a lot just by letting myself do what comes naturally.

No one wants to hear about motherly instincts. I wanted to rage against anyone who would bring up such a concept when I had my first baby. How was I supposed to have motherly instincts when I had just become a mother? Who had come up with this? What was wrong with me that I didn't know what to do?

Nothing was wrong with me. I just wasn't able to trust that I could live my way into the next moment instead of analyzing my way ahead of it. Much of the work of caring for babies and young children is not about rational thinking. I can read all the books I like and listen to all the experts, but unless I have Super Nanny living in my house 24-7, no one else will be able to give me an answer to each and every question I have. There is no flow chart to solve all the issues I will encounter. This can be incredibly frustrating to someone who is used to being able to think first, act next.

If, instead, I let myself respond to life naturally and witness my actions as they occur, I find greater access to intuition. Following the path of my natural tendencies, the answers I need seem to arise as I go along. As I mentioned before, I was recently offered a job. It wasn't just any job. It was an opportunity for flexible, part-time, meaningful work in a convenient location with a boss I already knew and really liked. Sounds like a no-brainer, right? But the decision wasn't that easy for me, the over-thinker, because every corner of my mind had to be searched for possible problems with the idea. When I eventually tired of the mental calisthenics, I slowed down and just observed my internal process. What I noticed was this: I felt scared.

Scared I wouldn't be able to find a trustworthy nanny for my eight-month-old baby and three-year-old son on such short notice.

Scared I would see even less of my five-year-old, who I already felt more separated from since he began elementary school.

Scared I wouldn't like the job but would be stuck in it because I felt a loyalty to my boss.

Scared I would feel overburdened, trying to manage work and three very young children.

Scared I would lose the shred of personal time I already had.

Scared of change.

But no, those were still just thoughts. The truth is, I felt scared. Period. So, the next step was to say, "Okay, Julia, you feel scared. Let's just feel scared now. Never mind the rationalizing of why you feel scared, and don't concern yourself with doing anything about it, not just yet." I stayed with the scared feeling to see where it took me. I just felt scared for a while.

When I let myself thoroughly feel my fear like this, it begins to dissolve. I get bored of being afraid and move on to other emotions. My mind still races, but so what? It just wants to know what happens next. It likes to solve problems and devise solutions to alleviate the fears. My heart can make the bigger choices, if I just move through what I feel.

So, in this situation, I felt afraid, and then I watched to see what would happen next. What happened next was this: I kept moving forward on the opportunity. Instead of arguing pros and cons, I started resolving logistics. I looked into childcare options, still feeling ambivalent and scared, but letting those feelings be part of the experience. Within two weeks time, a trusted friend had agreed to be our first nanny, and I started the new position.

In truth, I was always going to take that job. My fears were not going to stop me because it was too good of an opportunity to let pass. Sometimes, I go through the mental rigmarole of doubt, making things harder than they have to be. When instead I pay attention to my natural tendencies and internal leanings, I see that some part of me already knows where it wants to go.

Julia S. Aziz

Playfulness

I got into the shower and let the hot water soothe my aching back and tight belly. I danced and swayed through the contractions, spelling out words like "beautiful" and "open" and "trust." By repeating these words, I started to actually feel them. I wasn't exactly enjoying the contractions, but I was playing through them. Who could have imagined this peace in the midst of pain?

Life is easier when I am playful.

I live with one of the greatest teachers of playfulness. She is currently two and a half years old, and she is my daughter. My daughter finds fun wherever she goes. If there isn't already some fun waiting for her, she makes it. Through watching her, I learn the lesson of playfulness daily.

Every afternoon, when I pick up my daughter from her childcare program, she rushes to a couple of old poles that act as support beams for the carport. She puts one hand on the pole and throws the other to the wind, swinging herself around in circles. She twirls and swirls, smiling, until a friend comes outside and joins her on the other pole. Once they are together, my daughter laughs and laughs as she circles the pole. The first time this happened, the laughter came spontaneously. Now, she manufactures it, but just to get it started. She starts laughing, and then her friend will laugh, too.

Together, they keep swinging around the poles, laughing, until their forced laughter transforms into true giggling and squealing and they collapse into dizzy piles on the ground.

I love to watch my daughter spin even though I am often eager to get home by that time in the afternoon. Usually, I am tired, hungry, and desperate to get a few things done before my sons get home from school an hour later. Nonetheless, I watch her spin and marvel at how she makes the experience more fun by being playful with her friend. When I am really ready to leave, my best bet is to be playful right back with her. If I try to bargain, cajole, or force her into the car, she often ends up in tears, and I end up struggling to get her in the car seat. On the other hand, when I playfully threaten to "scoop her," she laughs maniacally and runs. She runs until I scoop her up sideways or upside down in my arms, wildly enough to make her squeal in delight. Together we laugh until, the next thing she knows, she is buckled into the car seat and we are on our way home.

My daughter was teaching me playfulness even from the womb, it seems. When I was pregnant with her, I started wearing lots of purple and pink. It wasn't because I anticipated having a girl baby; it was because I felt inspired to revive my own youthful and feminine nature. When I was about eight months pregnant, my friends hosted a mother's blessing for me. I had enjoyed a similar ritual near the end of each of my pregnancies, but this one was a little different. Instead of divulging my deepest fears about giving birth, I used the time to celebrate and play with my friends. We shared poems and blessings like we had in the earlier rituals, but this time we wore handmade butterfly barrettes and flowery dresses. Back at home later, my husband painted henna designs on my belly, and the boys took turns singing into my lap.

As I approached my due date, I wasn't concerned with all the physical symptoms of late pregnancy. I was already familiar with the hip pain, heartburn, and insomnia, and I didn't give those sensations much conscious attention. I just enjoyed being pregnant and everything that came with it: wearing loose dresses, feeling my baby move, and chatting with the strangers who wanted to touch my belly. I had fun with being nine months pregnant for the last time, and that made the experience seem a whole lot easier.

Julia S. Aziz

Flexibility

I started to wonder if I might be in transition, but dismissed the thought. It had been only ten minutes since we had determined that I was in active labor and called the midwife to come over. Then, my body started getting down on all fours in the narrow shower stall. I say "my body" did this because it was as if my mind was a witness to an unbelievable show. I just wasn't sure what I was watching. If I hadn't felt any pure soul-crushing pain, how could it be? But it was true, I realized then. My body was pushing the baby out, right there in my little shower. It was all happening now, with my husband at the other end of the house, unaware of my situation, and my midwife not yet with us.

I quickly found the presence of mind to leave. The shower stall was too small and slippery a space to give birth by myself. I turned off the water, grabbed my towel, and headed for the dining room. I found my husband reading the instructions on how to properly protect our futon mattress and sorting out the contents of the homebirth kit. Dripping wet, I told him I needed to get on that mattress ASAP even though it was at the moment covered in kitchen garbage bags (the plastic mattress protector having not yet been found). I told him I was pushing the baby out now and needed to get down on all fours. He was somewhat bewildered since just ten minutes before I had told him that I was "probably" in active labor. I got down on the mattress, and my water promptly broke. When I told my husband that the baby was coming out, he looked and concurred; he could see her head crowning. He was calm and supportive, with an "O.K., go ahead, we can do this," kind of attitude. I told him he would have to catch the baby, and he seemed unfazed. He got down behind me, remembering what he had learned from watching my other births, and called the midwife for guidance.

When faced with the unexpected, I can adapt and be flexible.

Being able to respond to circumstances with flexibility is a skill well worth cultivating. The more rigid I am about things going a certain way, the more trouble I get into. One of the greatest lessons of motherhood for me has been learning to bend as circumstances necessitate. When my first child skipped a nap, I would get frustrated about having to give up my alone time (needed for things like eating, showering, sleeping, not to mention anything beyond basic needs). Now, with three children, I see a long nap as a sort of surprise gift, and I have learned (mostly) to see the unexpectedness of my day as a challenge to be flexible.

This morning, for instance, after an hour of coaxing, my baby finally fell asleep. I had expected that we would have time for both a nap and a walk before we would need to pick up my son from preschool, but the settling down took longer than expected. I let the baby sleep for 40 minutes and then woke her up so that we could take a shorter but faster walk. On the way to the trail, it started to rain. I realized I had a choice. I could get frustrated about my morning, or I could just be flexible. I chose the latter and decided that we would do the walk in the rain, using an old sweatshirt for cover. It wasn't too cold out, and I love a good walk in the rain anyway. The baby won't melt—so why not?

Lessons of Labor

I have often said that the one quality I most hope for my children to possess is adaptability. I cannot pave their way in the world, but if they can be flexible and adjust to changing circumstances, I feel like they will be okay in the long run. Part of why I value flexibility so much for my children is because I know I need to develop it more for myself. So, I am working on it, bending and stretching all the time in response to the continuously surprising challenges that are thrown my way.

Julia S. Aziz

That Old Friend, Worry

*At that moment, the reality of the situation hit my brain.
Up until then, I had been letting my body lead. I was just
watching it and trying to understand. The pain was still manageable, not nearly as strong as it had been with the other two
labors. But there I was, crouching over a messy mattress on
my dining room floor with the baby crowning and the midwife
still on her way. Something clicked in my brain, reminding me
of the help I had needed when my sons were born. I remembered how my first son had to be suctioned and given oxygen in the hospital's intensive care unit right after his birth.
I remembered when my second son had gotten his shoulder
stuck and turned blue, and that the midwife had to coach me
through a non-contraction push at the last moment. Fear hit.
"I don't want to do this on our own. I want the midwife to be
here. I'm scared."*

*The fear I felt in those few minutes was clearly not coming
from my intuition. Everything had been moving so smoothly
and quickly ever since my day had quieted down. I didn't feel
like anything was wrong, but my mind started racing with
concerns: "My cervix has never been checked (not even during pregnancy)! The baby's heart rate has never been checked!
What about her position—is she in the right position? How do
I know she is okay in there?" Fast visions of my husband and
me delivering a stillborn baby raced through my head. Yet,*

my body felt like it was doing exactly what it needed to do. It was like my mind was playing an old movie, the old "birth fears" movie, and I just had to watch it one more time.

Just then, my friend Louise walked in the door with book and blanket in hand, expecting to go to sleep at our house like we had talked about less than an hour before. She quickly assessed that the situation had changed since I had called her. She asked what she could do, and I asked her to grab the camera. There was nothing else anyone could *do, except catch the baby. I saw the truth of this moment, and the worry subsided.*

Worry does not protect me from harm.

As I come from New York Jews on both sides, let me tell you, this lesson is one I am constantly relearning. I know quite a bit about worry, and I have consciously worked on releasing my belief in its benefit.

When my oldest son was four years old, he caught giardia, a parasite that causes six weeks of diarrhea and cramping. It took several weeks to diagnose the problem and to get a prescription for Flagyl to treat it. At the time, we were selling our home and buying a new house within a two month time frame. Life felt demanding and full. One day, while I was working on some mortgage paperwork, my son crawled into the bedroom. Confused and expecting some malingering for more attention, I asked him why he wasn't walking. He couldn't, he insisted. When I went to check on him, I realized that this was no joke. For some reason, he could not straighten his legs or put weight on his feet. By the time I got him to the doctor's office, twenty minutes later, he couldn't open his hands and had developed a fever and a rash all over his body. The doctor gave him Benadryl, explained that swelling was causing his inability to move, and said she wouldn't know the cause of the swelling until the lab tests came back.

Lessons of Labor

For about two weeks, our son gave lots of blood for various lab tests and saw allergy and rheumatology specialists. We were told he might have a chronic health issue like juvenile rheumatoid arthritis or lupus, but the results were still inconclusive. Every morning, he would run around as usual, but by the afternoon, he was immobilized. We would have to feed him with a spoon and carry him to the toilet because his hands and feet hurt so much. Later, the diagnosis came in that he was probably severely allergic to Flagyl, the medication that had been treating the giardia. Once the Flagyl fully left his system, he began to heal.

For those two weeks while we waited for an answer, no one knew how serious a health issue this would become. The uncertainty about my son's health, the extreme care he needed, and the continued house buying and selling negotiations threatened to drown me in worry. Maybe it was because there was too much to take in at the time, but I was able to find respite from the distress when I became conscious of it. There was too much to do to waste time thinking about how much worse things could get.

I remember thinking on that first drive to the doctor's office that something was really wrong this time but that my son would be okay. A lucky guess? Mother's intuition? Wishful thinking? Who knows, but sometimes I *do* know. Worry is just a distraction from that knowing and a stressful one at that. Even if my son had been diagnosed with a lifelong condition, worrying would not have offered comfort or solutions. It is just a habit of mind, and it does not have the power to save me or my loved ones. The less I believe and engage in worry, the more mental energy I can give to what is realistically within my power and capacity.

Julia S. Aziz

Competence and Ease

I started mentally repeating a request to my unborn daughter: "Just hold on until the midwife gets here, and then you can come right out." The pain of pushing, that now familiar ring of fire, barely registered in my brain. I was only focused on holding my baby in until professional help arrived. I didn't fight or try to control the pushing, but I didn't help it along. I just took shallow, panting breaths, let my body do its work, and asked my baby to come slowly.

Just a few minutes later, at 11:30 p.m., my midwife walked in the open door. She came straight over to me, crouched down, and caught my baby as she slipped easily out of my body.

Committing to the moment, I can discover competence and ease.

Do you know the feeling of being in the zone, when everything seems to fall into place with little or no effort? The freedom of living life in a state of flow is like no other I have known. While I may never achieve a level of mastery over parenthood, I do have moments of easy competence. I can look around and see that we are all doing pretty well.

Some Wednesday night last year, I was feeling a little dispirited and fatigued after a long day of work and parenting. While not an unusual scenario, this one stands out. On this particular Wednesday night, I impulsively decided to go to a free-form dance gathering that happens regularly in Austin. The idea came to me late, as it was already close to 9 p.m. and the music would end by 10 p.m. I hurried to get dressed and ran into my oldest son, who was having trouble sleeping. On a whim, I asked him if he wanted to come with me. "Yes!" he shouted, tearing off his pajamas and putting his clothes back on in under a minute. He knew full well how unusual an opportunity he had been given. A post-bedtime outing without his brother and sister was rare.

We hopped into the car and arrived at the studio, happily surprised by the half-price late-entrance fee. We entered the dance space where a diverse group of very expressive adults were dancing wildly in total silence except for the music. My son jumped right in. He leaped, he ran, he spun, he salsa-ed. Sometimes, I danced with him, following his lead as we zoomed in and out and made figure eights around all the other dancers. Sometimes, we danced separately, each finding our own rhythm. It was pure joy to express myself alongside my son. I loved the movement, the freedom, and the playful connection with him. We were in the zone, together. When we came home, he gave me a big hug of gratitude and went straight to bed. It was easy.

I remember this night clearly because it represents the magic that can unfold when I relax into an easy competence with my children and give in to the dance.

Potential Unbound

As I cradled my new daughter beneath a covering of blankets, my body shivered in shock. It was just 40 minutes ago that I had admitted I was in true labor, and now my baby was here! I had birthed her almost completely on my own. The whole experience was unlike my other labors in so many ways: the ease of the whole day, my willingness to be alone in labor while taking care of two children, the waiting to ask for help until the very end, and then my ability to hold the baby in until the midwife arrived. Somehow, I had lived my way into a greater sense of trust and capability than I had ever before possessed. It was a great beginning to this next chapter of my life.

I can do so much more than I think I can.

We can't even begin to know what we are capable of. Our imagined limits serve only as obstacles to trying new things. I used to see myself as a somewhat fragile person. I caught viruses often and cried easily, and I thought that meant I was weak. Giving birth allowed me to see my own strength, not just because I birthed a baby naturally but also because I had the tenacity and determination to continue in something that was hard.

While I loved nursing my babies, I also experienced ongoing breastfeeding issues. I saw multiple doctors, lactation consultants, and alternative healthcare professionals throughout my nursing years, and almost all of them eventually suggested I give up. They told me that some women just can't breastfeed and that I should accept that. Because I had plenty of milk to give and my babies were able to nurse, I was willing to withstand the recurrent pain and ruptured skin that afflicted me. Sometimes, it felt like I was pushing myself too hard, but other times, I saw the situation differently. As a homeopath once said to me, my willingness to suffer was remarkable. She didn't say this in a negative way but rather as an observation of my not backing down against great obstacles. Sure, call it stubborn. This stubbornness can impede flexibility, a quality necessary to a good life. It is also part of my strength.

It's important to realize that more is possible than I can now see. I used to look at other moms and wonder how some could do so much—work full-time in creative and meaningful jobs, cook elaborate and healthy meals, make time for their partner and friends, run marathons, and still parent with such patience and love. I now see that much of it is about believing in possibility. I practice thinking, "I can do this." I don't know how I'll do it, but if it's important, I will find a way. If I care about something wholeheartedly, I trust that the courage, the strength, and the energy will come when I need them.

MISCARRIAGE

The Birth of Unrealized Dreams
and Unexpected Tenderness

Julia S. Aziz

Embracing the Fragility of Life

A month after our wedding, I found out I was pregnant for the first time. I definitely wanted to have children relatively soon after getting married, but this pregnancy was not planned. We were hoping to buy a house, get a little more settled in our new jobs, and then begin this next stage of our lives. My husband and I were both incredulous and then overjoyed that I was pregnant so soon and so easily. A "wow, we really did this!" wonder and excitement coursed through me when we read the pregnancy stick after a couple weeks of sore breasts and a missed period. Immediately following the elation, a good dose of panic arrived. Should we still try to buy a house or just keep renting our small apartment? Would my new job offer maternity leave? Did I need a prenatal vitamin?

We decided to tell just one friend who had been pregnant recently. We knew we would need some advice and support but chose to wait before telling anyone else. Conventional wisdom said not to tell anyone in the first trimester, and we thought we should let the news sink in more, anyway.

As luck would have it, my husband and I were both beginning a winter break and were headed to south Texas for Christmas with his family. It was strange to hide such an exciting secret as we attended all the usual family gatherings, but we had a great Christmas day. I felt so thankful for all I had been given, especially my husband and this new baby.

My mind had finally settled down, and I was enjoying a new-found sense of connection and wellness.

Then, the next morning, the bleeding began. It started slowly but soon became voluminous. I was frightened, and I felt unnerved being in an unfamiliar city without my regular gynecologist. I asked the nurse on-call at my home doctor's office for advice, and she reassured me that while the process was very sad and painful, I was not in any danger. She was kind and understanding, and she walked me through what to expect and when to seek medical help. After getting off the phone, I felt slightly better but was still plagued with doubt. How could my body really lose this much blood so quickly? Why did it hurt so much? Despite the nurse's wise counsel, I went to the Emergency Room at the nearest hospital, convinced I needed some kind of intervention or assistance. After several hours of waiting, blood tests, and an ultrasound, it was confirmed that I had indeed been pregnant but would be no longer. My body was letting go, and the miscarriage was progressing naturally. It was over.

No one could tell me why I had lost this baby or what to do now that my pregnancy had ended. How could I let go of someone that never was? I was left with my questions and a profound sense of loss.

Life is so very fragile. Loss can happen in an instant; I will never see it coming. It leaves me with more questions than answers, and for a time, that is all I can take with me.

The things we have and the people we love in this lifetime, we will lose. Sometimes, it feels like there is no protection, knowing that everything can and will be taken away from me. In my good moments, I feel entirely liberated by that notion. If I can't hold on to anything, then I don't *need* to hold on to anything—I am free! However, in times of abrupt undoing, I am flooded with uncertainty and sorrow.

How can we absorb sudden loss? It is too much to take in all at once. The shock of how things can be one way and then be completely different is not digested by the mind or the body immediately. We have time, though. Just as the hours and days seemed to stretch on forever before the pivotal event, they will move slowly again in the time after.

When my children are in some kind of danger, there is absolutely nothing I wouldn't do to save them. However, most of the time they aren't in any danger other than the danger we all face in being mortal human beings. They were born into a life that will end in death someday. It is important, essential even, for me to remember that there is nothing I can do to change that. There is inherent risk in being alive, and even though we are resilient, we are also fragile. I can find the safest-seeming house in the safest-seeming neighborhood with the safest-seeming schools, but none of it comes with a guarantee. There is no easy prescription for how to live when we know our time together will end.

I knew from the moment I read the pregnancy test that miscarriage was a possibility. I never thought that it couldn't or wouldn't happen to me. Still, when it happened, I was in shock. The intensity of feeling nauseous all day and of reveling in my imaginary future was instantly replaced with an equal intensity of sadness, fear, and doubt. What could I learn from this loss, the loss of a life that ended before it even began? I carried this question with me in the weeks and months to come. At the time, there was no answer, just the question. At first, that is all we get.

Julia S. Aziz

Compassion

Devastated, we returned to our hotel room and called my family in upstate New York and my husband's family in town. It was heartbreaking to tell my mom our news in this way: "Mom, I was pregnant, but now I am miscarrying." She was immediately sympathetic. She, too, had miscarried a baby and knew instinctively the kind of compassionate holding I needed. My husband's family was supportive, too, bringing us take-out food and giving us space to grieve without the pressure to attend further holiday celebrations. My husband was right there with me, heavy with sadness and regret. We had each been through some difficult times when we dated, but this was the first loss we shared as a married couple. We had created and loved something together, and while the loss was unbelievably sad, it also brought us a new sense of unity and tenderness.

When I returned home, I told quite a few friends about what had happened. I needed to talk about it because it was all I could think about. What helped the most was talking to the few people I knew who had miscarried and the friends who were able to sit with my distress instead of dismissing it or solving it away. More than anything, I needed compassion.

When the heart loses, it also opens.

We hear that around 20% of pregnancies probably end in miscarriage, and most of us know at least a few women who have experienced them. Unless you have lost a baby yourself, though, it can be hard to understand. Even if you have experienced pregnancy loss, it may hold different meaning for you than it does for others. For this reason, people don't always know what to say or do when their loved one miscarries. It is usually a private grief, with no funeral and often not a lot of sympathy. "You can always try again," is a common refrain, and while this is often true and meant to be comforting, it doesn't recognize the genuine heartbreak.

For me, miscarriage meant the loss not only of a pregnancy but also the loss of an individual human being that never made it into the world. Too, it was the loss of an unrealized dream, one that my husband and I had imagined together. For almost two weeks, my body continued to bleed, constantly reminding me of my sorrow, while the still unanswered question of my fertility weighed on my heart. I felt like I had plunged into a deep darkness, into waters where I could barely keep afloat. I could not stop crying or stop thinking about this potential life that had ended so swiftly. Even after being momentarily distracted, I would quickly, almost purposefully, turn back toward my grief. It was all I had left of my baby, and I knew, with time, I wouldn't even have that sadness to hold onto anymore.

My heart was wide open, so vulnerable and so tender. I had to be careful about whom I talked to because I could so easily feel misunderstood or injured. I could have shut down from the world completely, but something in me needed connection. My heart needed to feel the love and support that was available, to reach out for the lifeline that would pull me out of the darkness.

In the periphery of my sadness, I was able to glimpse the compassion surrounding me. A dear friend had miscarried within a week of me, and she was my companion in grief over the long distance phone lines. My mom sent beautiful cards and phone messages. My husband was by my side, feeling everything. I also had some local friends who were patient and understanding, allowing me my darkness but inviting me to emerge when I was ready. I felt raw and exposed, grateful for the few people who knew how to open their hearts and be with that vulnerability without telling me, "It happens all the time. Of course, you will have another baby."

There are many women who have borne great losses. Some desperately want biological children but are unable to conceive them. Some give birth to babies who never take a single breath. Some lose living children. In comparison, a miscarriage is minor and commonplace, but comparing grief helps no one. The gift of my miscarriage was that it broke my heart open to a new level of compassion, and as a result, I vowed to reach out to women going through similar experiences. Sometimes, I have known these women intimately; sometimes, they have only been acquaintances. When I hear of a pregnancy loss, I try to let the mother know that she is not alone and that I am willing to listen if she needs someone.

A friend miscarried not long ago, and she, too, was deeply affected by it. I made sure to ask her how she was doing, not only right when it happened but also months later. From my own experience, I knew that just because the bleeding has stopped doesn't mean the grief has ended. I wanted to be available to her when the intensity had died down, when the period of acceptable mourning had passed, and when most people wanted her to move on. Before my own miscarriage, I still felt a lot of empathy toward women who had experienced pregnancy loss, whether they were my counseling clients or friends. Now, my heart is touched in a different way. This particular grief has given me a deeper level of understanding, and for that, I am thankful.

Julia S. Aziz

Patience With My Process

It took me a long time to "get over" the miscarriage. I spent days on end listening to the same sad songs on repeat, writing in my journal, and taking warm baths. The mourning seemed to linger on in a way that it hadn't for many of my friends and acquaintances who had lost pregnancies. Sometimes, I would wonder why I couldn't seem to move on the way they could. Over weeks and months, though, the wound began to heal, leaving an emotional scar just noticeable enough to remember.

Instead of getting pregnant right away and filling the hole that this baby had left, I grieved. In time, I could appreciate this slow path and the meaning I found in mourning.

There are no rules to grief, though we may try to impose them. What I need most is patience with my own process.

Cultures deal with grief differently. In the Judaism I was raised in, family and friends visit and pray together for seven days after a death, finding solace in a community of mourning. In the workaday American culture, many businesses offer a three day bereavement leave, but only if the person who died was an immediate family member. After that, it's back to work.

Life does need to go on, of course. We do need to continue our labors and our living. We cannot exist on hold forever, but despite what actions we need to take outwardly, the inner process of letting go takes its own time.

Before having children, I had the incredible experience of working for a home hospice organization as a spiritual counselor. It was truly an honor to work in such a role. My job was to visit dying people and their family members in their homes. I would talk, read, meditate, and pray, but mostly I listened. I listened to their nostalgia for the past, to their anger at disease, to their frustration with medical help, and to their disappointment in loved ones. I heard their stories of love and loss, and eventually I heard their fears, once they were ready to admit and accept what was inevitable.

Watching the hospice patients and family members, I learned the unique ways that people respond to the process of dying, which is also a process of grieving. When there is some time for awareness before death, there is an opportunity to grieve before the final hour arrives. What I noticed was that people tended to approach dying in the same way that they had approached living. Some of the hospice patients said their goodbyes soon after their diagnoses and readied themselves for the end. Others fought their way to their very last breath. Others would hold on for many months, even years, in a state of very little living, but not yet dying. These months and years were incredibly hard for their loved ones, but this time was necessary. It was the process they needed in order to let go.

How do we have patience with a process that is so uncomfortable and so slow that it seems like it will always stay the same? I think we can only live out that question in our hearts. We just live each day, feeling the sadness, the anger, the pain, and then somewhere down the line, it fades a little, then a little more. No matter what I do, this letting go takes its own time. Patience is what I really need.

Julia S. Aziz

Making Meaning

We named our lost baby Obie, a nickname for O.B., or Our Baby, which was what we had been calling him or her in utero. We found a place along our favorite hiking trail to bury some symbolic remains, carving the baby's name into a plank of wood next to a pond. The wood was part of a small dock that we were sure to visit again over the years. Later, I created a collage of mementos: my hospital bracelet from the Emergency Room visit, a condolence card, and some photos from those few weeks when I knew I was pregnant. I took pictures of the collage and placed them in our photo album, right after our wedding photos. These small rituals gave voice to my grief, a place for my sorrow.

Being creative in ritual brings me back to center and helps me find meaning.

Despite the many mourning rituals in different cultures and religions, there are very few for miscarriage in modern American life. Most women suffer silently until time allows them more space from their sadness. Time certainly is the most effective healer, but for me, it wasn't enough. I wanted a tangible way to say goodbye. I needed to release my attachment to this particular baby so that I could move on to welcoming the next. It was hard to mourn for Obie, not having a body that I could ever hold and not having a community that shared my loss. It was as if that short time of pregnancy was all a dream. I needed to know it was real to acknowledge that my feelings were real.

By creating ritual, I was able to mark this period in my life. By marking it, I could find closure to it. Through memorializing Obie and the love I felt, I was able to honor this baby and honor myself. I still look at the collage once in a while, and I always visit our makeshift memorial site when I walk on that trail. I take my children there to hike and climb trees; it is still my favorite park in Austin. When I rub my fingers along the carving of our long-ago baby's name, I remember my husband and me as we used to be. I remember our new marriage, the hope we began with, and the compelling desire to create a family out of our love. There is sweetness to the reminiscing now. Having a place where I am reminded of how we began is a touchstone for who we have become.

Allowing The Longing

Along with the sadness and the temptation to blame my-self (Should I have been traveling? Did I do something wrong?) was the fear that I would not be able to carry a pregnancy the next time we tried. I wanted a baby desperately. All of a sudden, the desire went from a nagging whisper to an urgent scream. We held off on trying to get pregnant again since we wanted to buy a house and take a long-awaited honeymoon first. I held my desire close to my heart for six months, acutely wanting to act but choosing not to.

I can allow my longing to exist without trying to fill it.

A month or so after the miscarriage, I visited a wise mentor. I told her how desperately I wanted a baby, how it felt like I could barely breathe, the longing was so strong. Instead of talking me out of my desire or helping me plan how to fulfill it, she suggested I befriend my yearning. She reminded me that women have yearned for babies throughout human history. This longing is part of our legacy. What comfort I took in that wisdom! What relief! I had been given permission to feel the intensity of my longing without the pressure to do anything about it.

Rationally, I knew that more stability would create more space in our lives for a child. It made sense to find a home to settle into, to give ourselves some time to enjoy being married, and to celebrate this brief child-free period in our marriage with a romantic and fun vacation. All these reasons added up to waiting another six months before trying to get pregnant. It wouldn't be very long to wait. By losing this baby, we had been given a chance to be more intentional about getting pregnant. We had a logical plan.

My heart didn't like it, though, and I had been trying to rationalize with my heart, to no avail. Taking my friend's advice, I started to just acknowledge the longing. I listened to the internal voice of desire without argument. I tried to offer compassion for the powerful urge to create and to love. I wrote pages and pages about how much I wanted a child, including all my fears, doubts, and impassioned pleas. I crafted some of this writing into an intention. That's what I called it, but maybe it was a wish or just something to speak to the universe. I sent this writing to my mentor so that she, too, could acknowledge and send love towards my longing.

I still waited the six months, and I still wanted to get pregnant right away. It was okay, just the way it was.

So often we try to fill the holes of desire. I try to satisfy a lack of purpose with socializing. I glaze over discomfort by watching television. These strategies do work, for a while. Surprisingly, it also works to just take a look in there, in that lonely and barren place where we await something that may never materialize. In that place, I see the beauty of longing, and I learn to live alongside it.

Gratitude

It sounds strange to say but even in the first weeks after my miscarriage, there was an intimation of gratitude. Despite my heartache, I was so thankful that I had been able to experience being pregnant. I didn't know what the future would hold, but I had really wanted to get pregnant someday. I had never been sure if I would be able to. This baby Obie taught me that I could conceive at a time when I really needed to know that. I wouldn't have chosen to lose the pregnancy, but I had, at least, been able to experience it. We only get one chance to experience something for the first time, and that may be the only chance we ever get. For that brief encounter with my dream, I was grateful.

When I think of Obie now, it is with a prayer of gratitude for his or her short presence in my life. He or she is the one who readied me for the biggest transformation I would ever know.

There is something to be grateful for in every experience of my life.

I cannot give thanks for losing an unborn baby because to do so would be to dishonor my grief and the short life of that struggling being. However, I do give thanks to Obie for introducing me to the deep devotion, anxiety, and determination of mother-love, which has made my life richer in so many ways. Even though I was not able to hold him or her

189

in my arms, that small baby in my womb inspired an attachment in me that I had never known before. Obie opened me to the possibility of motherhood, igniting a desire that had been there for years, probably. I had wanted children but had been afraid of the responsibility. After the miscarriage, those fears seemed insignificant. I knew it was time to take the leap, and I was ready. Because I lost Obie, I gained courage, enough to eventually have three children.

Obie also taught me about the potential for healing, for others as well as for myself. I was able to see that over the course of time my grief lessened and transformed itself into gratitude, a healing that I could not have imagined initially. The memory that remains is no longer painful; rather, it is a sacred and private scar I can share when another woman bears a similar loss.

If Obie had survived, the three particular children I now have would not be alive. Losing Obie paved the way for these incredible human beings who are growing healthy and strong every day. A few weeks ago, my younger son noticed a small Christmas stocking that I had placed near my meditation space. I explained to him about the baby that had started to grow in my belly but had never made it all the way into the world. I told him that this stocking was for Obie and that, in my heart, Obie was like a guardian angel for our family. He was part of us—part of our story and part of our love. Right away, my son understood. He has no barriers to imagination, no set rules about death. Together, we appreciated this little almost-life that had been with us at the very beginning.

Saying Goodbye, Moving Forward

Was it weeks or months before the loss felt less like a knife to the gut and more like a faint whisper of love? I do not know, though I do know that when I gave birth to my first son a year and a half later, something released in me that had been holding tight since I lost Obie. I was able to finally say goodbye when my new life as a mother began.

Birth is both beginning and ending.

The loss of a baby not yet ready to live in this world may be the most poignant example of birth as both beginning and ending. Women who have suffered through miscarriages, stillbirths, or babies that die within hours of being born can all attest to this. These births that are also deaths are too much to bear, and yet they must be endured. Mothers and fathers are forced to live on and begin anew, with grief as a companion and a reminder of lost love.

In a more metaphorical way, birth is always an end, even when it results in a happy and healthy baby ready to grow and thrive. A new mother often does not anticipate the grief she may feel for her old life, that independent existence where she made choices as a solo traveler upon the earth. I remember distinctly the first time I drove away from my first baby and how excruciating it was to leave him. My attachment to him was absolute, and he, such a fragile being, was dependent on me for his very survival. It felt simultaneously terrifying and completely normal to be out on my own. In truth, just a week before, I had been a child-free woman. The change was so dramatic that I had forgotten how recently it had occurred. Months later, I would cherish any moment I could spend alone, whether I was showering, driving to work, or grocery shopping. Now, eight years and three children later, I can intellectually recall the pre-motherhood freedom that I enjoyed, but it is not a visceral memory. For this particular phase of my life, solitude and independence are rare.

Our newborn babies, too, teach us about endings. In being born, they lose that intimate reliance on the mother's womb. Within months, they emerge so completely that we find it hard to believe they ever fit so neatly inside our bodies. The journey of pregnancy, so consuming while it occurs, is brief in retrospect.

Even when I already had a child, the births of my second and third children marked the end of different chapters. As we became a newly expanded family, we also said goodbye to the family we had been. As we grew in number, each child lost some individual attention from a parent; each parent lost some solo time with a child. These endings were worth the new love that arrived, but in all the beauty of new beginnings, it is easy to forget the little losses along the way.

When I choose to honor both the beginnings and the endings in my life, I am filled with reverence. I am grateful to be a part of this world that includes both new creation and loss. Knowing such beautiful joy and sorrow, I remember what it truly means to live.

Afterword

It's all so different than I thought it would be.

A new friend spoke these words above about motherhood, and I agree completely. My life as a new mother was different than I imagined it would be, and as my children grow, I continue to be surprised.

Nothing can truly prepare you for birthing or for motherhood because it is new territory. Your life will not be the same, and while you may have seen this transformation happening for other women, there is no way to know how having a child will change you. I say this not to be dramatic but to relieve the burden of needing to know something that can't be known.

Birth is the transition, the final words of the chapter and the preface to the next, all at once. It is how we mark time, and it is to be celebrated and deeply honored.

If I had to say some final words to a new mom, they would be this: trust and be kind to yourself. If you can do these things as often as possible, you will, I believe, do a great job taking care of your babies.

May we birthe and mother as we wish to live, in peace and in awe of all that life is.

Julia S. Aziz

Acknowledgements

There are many friends and family members who have supported me through this decade of early motherhood. They are part of my story, as I am a part of theirs. I am grateful for the many kind words, the long walks, the babysitting, the meals, the hand-me-downs, the girls' nights, the playdates, the camping trips, the laughter, and the time together. I thank every one of these beautiful people for accompanying me on this journey.

Additionally, I would like to acknowledge those who have played indispensable roles in the birth of this book.

I am grateful to the wonderful midwives who helped me give birth: Meredith Klein, Mary Barnett, Siobhan Kubesh, and Julia Bower. Their trust in the body and the birthing process has inspired me on so many different levels.

I am grateful to Betty Lou Leaver at MSI Press for seeing the potential in a rough labor of love. Her guidance gave me just the impetus I needed to pull it all together.

I am grateful to Carly Willsie for publishing advice and for reminding me why I wanted to allow these words into the world in the first place. I wish her incredible joy as she makes her own transformation into motherhood now.

I am grateful to those friends who were willing to read this manuscript in its early stages. I thank Jill Davis for being my very first reader and Megan Barnes Zesati for her constructive feedback. I am also especially grateful to Sarah Sullivan and Shawna Weekly for encouragement when my inner critics were stomping about.

I am grateful to the South Austin women's career circle (or whatever we want to call it) for standing by me, holding me accountable, and egging me on.

I am grateful to my mom, Betty Zimmerberg, for setting the example of incredible natural birthing and for the countless ways she has shown her love for our growing family.

I am grateful to my dad, Stanley Glick, for believing in this book so immediately and unconditionally.

I am deeply grateful to my husband, Patrick Aziz, without whom none of this would have happened. Not only would I not have our children without him, I would not have this book, either. Because he stepped up so tirelessly and without complaint to take care of our children while I wrote, this book was finished. I thank him for believing in me, encouraging me, and standing by my side as a writer, as a partner, and as a person. I look forward to many more years of learning and loving together.

I am beyond grateful to my children, Kaleb, Jeremiah, and Marisa Aziz. They were patient with my absences while I wrote and always greeted me with big hugs when I returned. I hope someday when they read these stories that they know I don't regret a single moment. While I share a lot of my struggles in this book, there are so many easy, happy times that are not included. I am honored to be the mother of such amazing individuals, and I love them with a devotion that cannot be measured. I thank all three of them for teaching me so much about kindness, receptivity, healing, joy, and above all, love.

Lastly, I offer profound gratitude to the infinite mystery of it all, the big unknowable pattern of which I am just one small spark, for this lifetime of learning.

Julia S. Aziz

Selected Publications of MSI Press

365 Teacher Secrets for Parents: Fun Ways to Help Your Child Succeed in Elementary School (McKinley & Trombly)

A Believer-in-Waiting's First Encounters with God (Mahlou)

Blest Atheist (Mahlou)

Creative Aging (Vassiliadis & Romer)

Forget the Goal; the Journey Counts. . . 71 Jobs Later (Stites)

How To Be a Good Mommy When You're Sick: A Guide to Motherhood with Chronic Illness (Graves)

It Only Hurts When I Can't Run (Parker)

Losing My Voice and Finding Another (Thompson)

Mommy Poisoned Our House Guest (S. Leaver)

Of God, Rattlesnakes, and Okra (Easterling)

Syrian Folktales (M. Imady)

Publishing for Smarties: Finding a Publisher (Ham)

The Gospel of Damascus (O. Imady)

The Marriage Whisperer: Tips to Improve Your Marriage Overnight (Patt Pickett)

The Road to Damascus (E. Imady)

Thoughts without a Title (Henderson)

CPSIA information can be obtained
at www.ICGtesting.com
Printed in the USA
BVOW11s2210020616

450480BV00009B/79/P